A Doctor for the People

A Doctor for the People

2000 years of general practice in Britain

John Cule MA, MD, FRCGP

Fellow of the Faculty of the History and Philosophy of Medicine and Pharmacy of the Worshipful Society of Apothecaries of London; Lecturer in the History of Medicine, Welsh National School of Medicine.

1980
Update Books
London/Dordrecht/Boston

Available in the UK and Eire from:
Update Books Ltd.,
33–34 Alfred Place, London WCIE 7DP, England.

Available in the USA and Canada from:
Kluwer Boston Inc.,
Lincoln Building, 160 Old Derby St., Hingham, Mass. 02043, USA.

Available in the rest of the world from:
Kluwer Academic Publishers Group,
Distribution Centre, PO Box 322, 3300 AH Dordrecht, The Netherlands.

British Library Cataloguing in Publication Data

Cule, John
  A Doctor for the people
  1. Family medicine—Great Britain
  —History
  I. Title
  362.1'0425   R729.5.G4
ISBN-13: 978-94-011-6388-0   e-ISBN-13: 978-94-011-6386-6
DOI: 10.1007/978-94-011-6386-6

ISBN-13: 978-94-011-6388-0

Designed by: Viv Wilcock, SIAD, STD

Typeset and produced by: R. James Hall
Typesetting & Book Production Services
Harpenden, England

Type face: Garamond 11pt on 12.

Printed through Hans Blaauw by
Drukkerij Groen IJmuiden bv
The Netherlands

First published 1980
© Update Books Ltd. 1980
Softcover reprint of the hardcover 1st edition 1980

Contents

Contents

Preface

This book has been written to show how the personal medical care of the patient began and was later shaped by cultural, political and scientific changes in Britain. It is, therefore, the story of the evolution of the general medical practitioner as we know him today.

The history of general practice is largely the history of medicine. Politicians have commented that there are as many different concepts of general practice as there are general practitioners. On the other hand, as many types of general practice are demanded by patients as there are types of patient. Yet a common thread runs through the whole of general practice: the supply of a skilled medical service to all those who need it, at all times.

The book is by no means a comprehensive study and is meant for doctors and patients, as well as medical and social historians who are interested in the history of general practice in Britain. Many people not directly connected with the practice of medicine have attended the teaching course organised by the Worshipful Society of Apothecaries of London for their Diploma of the History of Medicine, and the idea for this book grew out of my lectures on that course. As it is meant as a general introduction, outlining the changing face of medicine, I have indicated books for further reading, rather than burden the text with detailed source references.

I am indebted to many people for making this book possible. The help of librarians, particularly Mr Eric Freeman of the Wellcome Institute for the History of Medicine, has been invaluable. In the preparation for press, Miss Ann Thorneywork, Assistant to the Editor of Update Books, has been an indefatigable searcher for illustrations, and I have had the skilful guidance of Mrs Maggie Pettifer, Editor of Update Books.

John Cule
Llandysul
July 1980

1
Pre-Roman Britain

The origins of general medical practice extend far beyond the history of the modern type of general medical practitioner. In Britain, personal medical care can be traced to pre-Roman times. Medical ideas in other countries have also influenced its development and lead us firstly to a brief general look at the evidence of ancient illness and medical practice overseas as well as at home, before considering in particular the recorded shape of early medical care in Britain.

The lack of written sources is a major problem in searching for the beginnings of medical practice. Fortunately, palaeopathologists, studying the disease processes in bodies preserved from ancient times, as well as anthropologists, studying social behaviour in contemporary and historical societies, have helped to fill the gap. One example of such evidence is the discovery of fractured bones showing callus formation. From these we can learn the type of injuries that people received and whether or not they recovered from them. Yet there are obvious dangers in using such non-written testimony to establish the quality of man's existence. It should not be assumed that a bone which has healed successfully indicates intentional human therapy. R. L. Moodie, the American anatomist who in 1923 published the first comprehensive book on palaeopathology, records callus in the fractured radius of a Permian reptile that died 250 million years ago!

Diseases and Medical Treatment in Early Civilisations

INFECTIONS FROM PALAEOLITHIC TO MESOLITHIC TIMES

Don R. Brothwell, an eminent contemporary anthropologist with a great interest in palaeopathology, quotes Hare's view that 'the less harmful commensals such as the staphylococci of the skin, the streptococci of the throat, and the coliform organisms of the bowel are likely to be older than man, and just as likely then as now to give rise to inflammatory conditions of the tissues'. Most communities had to rely on the healing processes of nature in the

1. Femur and scurvy changes.
Photographed by Hallam Ashley.
By courtesy of the Norfolk Museums Service.

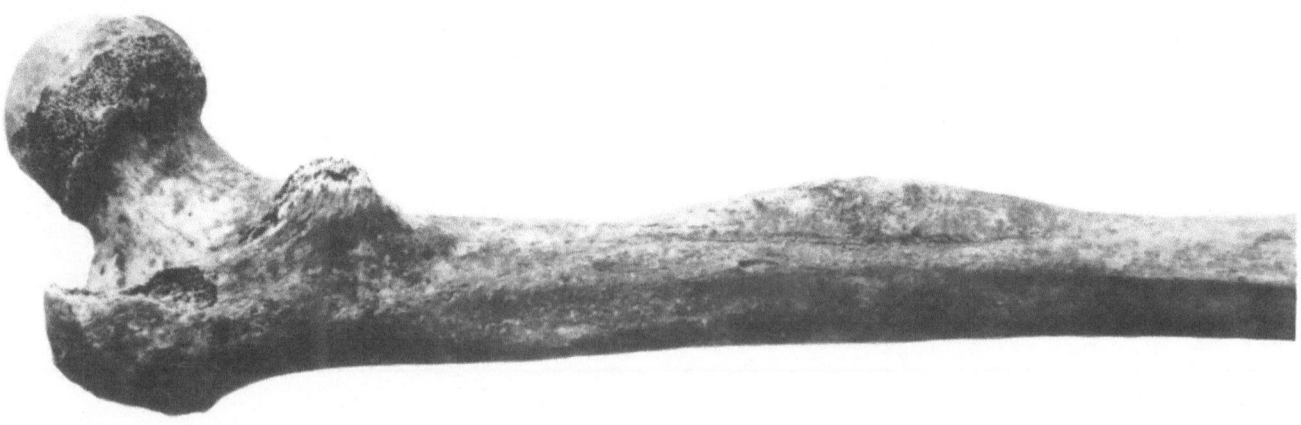

recovery from these diseases. Indeed it is possible that many of the bacteria that we regard as harmless today, might have been severely pathogenic in earlier times. Highly virulent organisms infecting small susceptible communities not only destroyed their hosts, but in so doing ultimately destroyed themselves by removing their stores for future nutriment. It was only after attenuation of their own virulence that they continued to flourish. Thus the majority of the hunters and food gatherers of Palaeolithic and Mesolithic times would have been wiped out in an epidemic, leaving behind very few to acquire much immunity. Not until the Neolithic Revolution and the resulting increase in size of the agricultural communities was the scene set for the proliferation of disease, and the development of immunity.

THE WORK OF THE PALAEOPATHOLOGISTS

Palaeopathologists have given us some insight into the type of diseases people suffered from (figure 1), yet their conclusions are largely speculative. Dr Calvin Wells reported an early Bronze Age skeleton from Norfolk with an atrophy of the long bones of one arm:

It is a reasonable conjecture to suppose that the markedly lighter build of this left arm is the result of a disuse atrophy. If so there can be little doubt that poliomyelitis occurring in adolescence or early adult life would be the most likely cause of it although other conditions such as Erb's paralysis cannot be excluded with absolute certainty.

Nor indeed can any other form of nerve injury or disease be dismissed.

There is a well known deformity of the left foot in the mummy of the Pharaoh Siphtah (XIXth Dynasty) which Elliot Smith attributed to poliomyelitis. An even earlier example, illustrated in Sigerist's *Primitive and Archaic Medicine* of an XVIIIth Dynasty stele, depicts an atrophied right leg with a talipes equinus that might have resulted from an attack of the same disease.

Degenerative diseases, such as osteoarthritis, and the ever present problem of dental caries have been in Britain since at least Neolithic times. Bones and teeth, which are the most enduring parts of the human frame show evidence of osteitis and abscess formation. Some authorities have attempted even more definitive diagnoses such as osteomyelitis and bone tuberculosis. My colleague Lynn Evans and I, after studying the sixteenth century BC Gelligaer skull of a Bronze Age child were only able to reach the conclusion that some of the bone changes could have been caused by a severe anaemia. This might have been aggravated by two attacks of some infection, for there are two clear horizontal grooves in the enamel of the left upper permanent canine tooth caused by the disturbances of growth at these times. The probability of a deficiency anaemia in a Bronze Age child, living in the Welsh hills, must have been considerable, without even the hope of supplementary benefit from iron food utensils!

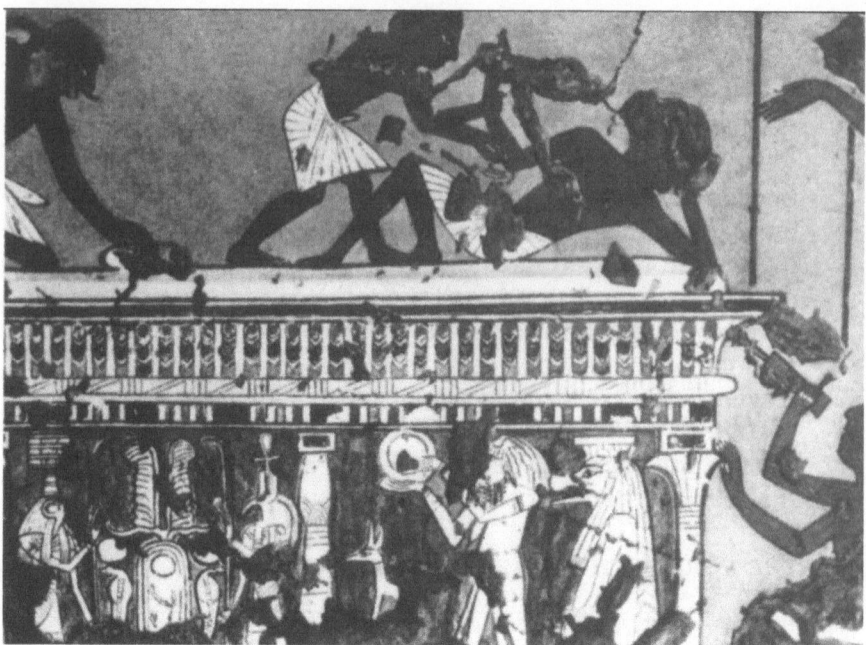

2. A painting of an Egyptian doctor setting a dislocated shoulder on a building site.
By courtesy of the Metropolitan Museum of Arts, New York.

EARLY RECORDS OF MEDICAL TREATMENT

The Edwin Smith Papyrus, written about 1600 BC, is itself probably a copy of a surgical text which could have been written a thousand years earlier in the Pyramid Age. Although it deals with the diagnosis of fractures and their treatment by reduction and splinting there is no evidence that this knowledge was available in Europe until the time of Hippocrates in the fifth century BC, and not in Britain until the time of the Romans. The same Egyptian manuscript deals with the treatment of wounds, but doubtless many injuries of varying degrees of severity healed with varying degrees of success, both in Egypt and Britain, without the aid of early surgical science (figure 2).

Societies in Pre-Roman Britain

THE POPULATION OF PRE-ROMAN BRITAIN

The population of Britain was very small: it varied from a few hundred in Palaeolithic times to a few thousand in the Neolithic age. Piggott, in *Ancient Europe*, makes a reasoned guess that the population south of the limit of permanent ice in Late Glacial Britain might have been 250, in roughly 10 hunting groups of 20 to 25 people. By analogy with Australian aborigines or Caribou eskimos, the density could be expected to be about three persons per hundred square miles. The total of 250 humans may be on the low side, but the highest possible figure is likely to be no more than 2,000. After 8000 BC, the last of the final glacial phases was over, and Piggott estimates that the population of Britain might have reached 10,000 persons by the year 7500 BC. Fleure, in his book *Natural History of Man in Britain*, conjectures that by Neolithic times, with a more settled and growing population, and probably a fall in infant mortality, the womenfolk would have had to bear an average of six children each to keep the population from

4

decreasing. In the second millenium, the population might have reached 100,000.

The first agriculturists were establishing themselves in Britain before 3000 BC and the transition from the hunting and food gathering stage to that of deliberate food production had begun. With the domestication of animals and the cultivation of crops, the scene was set for a more settled existence and a life of greater certainty. Next to nothing is known of their social organisation.

There is evidence of technological development in the cultures of the Bronze Age and the Iron Age, and of their burial customs in those of the Megalith builders and the Beaker folk. Metal objects, pots, shards, cists and barrows reveal the early presence of man, by these recognisably human pursuits. The archaeologist uncovers traces of communities with characteristics that we can acknowledge as similar to our own, and with a desire to do more than simply to survive. Ornaments were made and pots were decorated to provide beauty as well as utility. In such groups there was probably a religion. For any surmise of their social behaviour, one has to rely on the work of the social anthropologists as there is no written evidence.

THE PROBLEMS OF USING NON-WRITTEN EVIDENCE

There are dangers in making analogies between the early societies of pre-history and the primitive societies of today. In comparison with modern advanced societies, the primitive communities have a very basic social structure, and a simple economy, with little specialisation in jobs. Evans Pritchard comments in his book *Social Anthropology*, that as far as we know, 'primitive societies may have just as long a history as our own, and while they are less developed in some respects they are often more developed in others'. One can also sympathise with Graham Clark's aphorism, 'to the peoples of the world generally . . . I venture to think that Palaeolithic Man has more meaning than the Greeks'.

In the absence of any written evidence about the earliest communities, one has to rely on analogy and the reconstructions made by social anthropologists. There is universal evidence in support of the constancy of human nature shown by the similarity of human ideas and the changelessness of human behaviour which has emerged independently from differing geographical sites throughout the ages.

Anthropologists have studied the customs, oral traditions, technology, art, social structure and religious beliefs in modern primitive societies. These studies have provided information about their care of the sick and we can try by analogy to understand their counterparts in the societies of pre-history.

CARE OF THE SICK IN PRIMITIVE SOCIETIES

Medical care began within the family: women looked after their children and their men, and learnt, for example, that bleeding could be staunched by pressure from the hand and that thorns and parasites could be extracted with the fingers. They treated these minor ailments with simple domestic remedies, and those who became particularly skilful at it were increasingly in demand as the communities grew. Sigerist states that these simple ailments did not bestow on the sufferer a special position in society, 'they are treated with domestic remedies and disappear, as they came, without requiring an explanation and without preventing the patient from sharing in the life of the group'.

Serious disease, which prevented the sufferer from taking his share in the tasks required of him, differentiated him from the rest of the tribe. His fate then depended on the basic nature of the economy. It was economically necessary to kill members of the nomadic hunting and food gathering groups, once they were incapable of carrying out their duties. The cannibal societies killed and ate those who were no longer of any use to the community, and this they did as soon as possible, before the victims had lost too much weight. The economy of the later static agricultural societies allowed them to take a more liberal attitude toward those who were ill, and attempt to provide them with medical care.

Rituals in Diagnosis and Treatment

PRIMITIVE CONCEPTS OF DISEASE

The societies of pre-Roman Britain, who knew nothing about the real cause of disease, accounted for such misfortune in the same way that they explained any other natural disaster. Chance was not an acceptable explanation. As jealousy or avarice often motivated men to destroy each others' crops and animals, so floods and droughts could be caused by spirits who had been displeased. Many of the spirits were thought to be those of the ordinary dead, while many of the ruling spirits were believed to be those of dead great men. Sometimes inanimate objects also had spirits, but the concept was always that each had a personality and, as with human beings and consequently human spirits, could be both offended and appeased.

It thus was logical for these people to accept the abnormal condition of patients suffering from serious diseases, as the effect of transcendental forces that had gained power over them. They believed that illness was caused by an external spiritual, rather than an internal physical cause.

THE WORK OF THE PRACTITIONERS

It therefore followed that a practitioner, expert on the nature of spiritual interference, had to establish the cause of an illness before he could advise on an appropriate remedy. He had to decide whether the spirits had been offended by the transgression of a taboo, been invoked by the malice of an enemy, or provoked by the deliberate disobedience of the patient. In order to do this, a

6

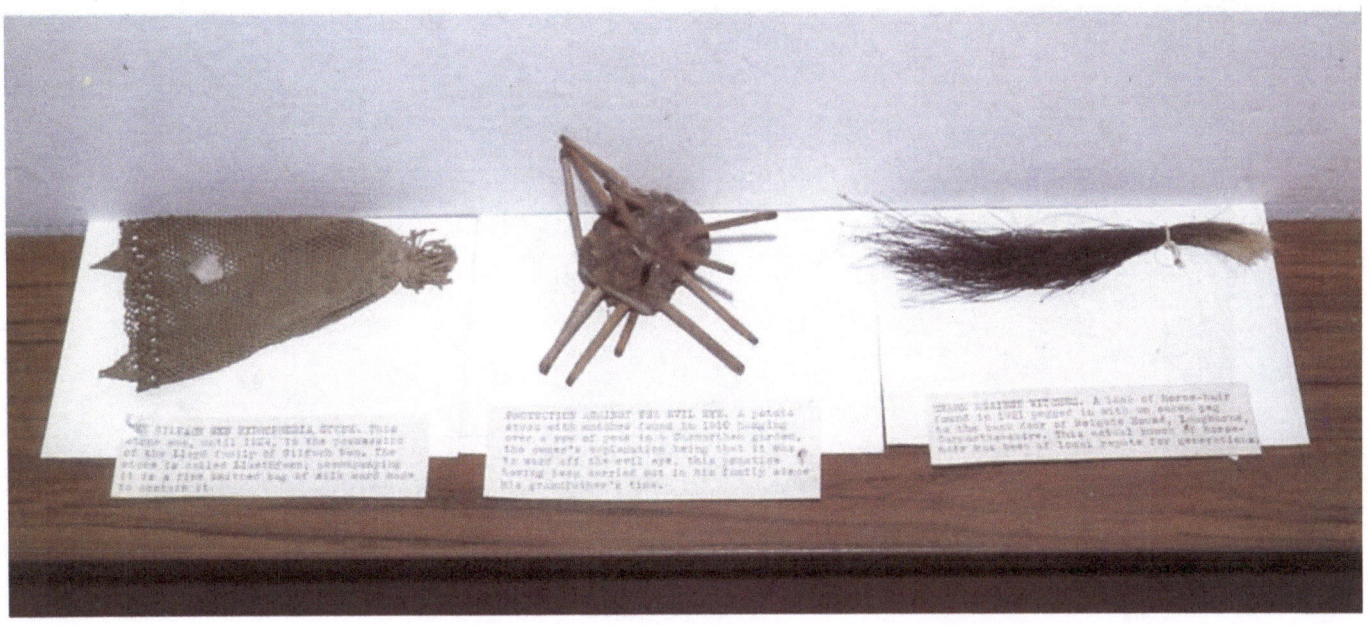

III
Charms against witches. A lock of
horse hair found in 1921, pegged with
an oaken peg to the back door of a
house in Laugharne, Carmarthenshire.
This actual bunch of horse hair had
been of local repute for generations.
By courtesy of Carmarthen Museum.

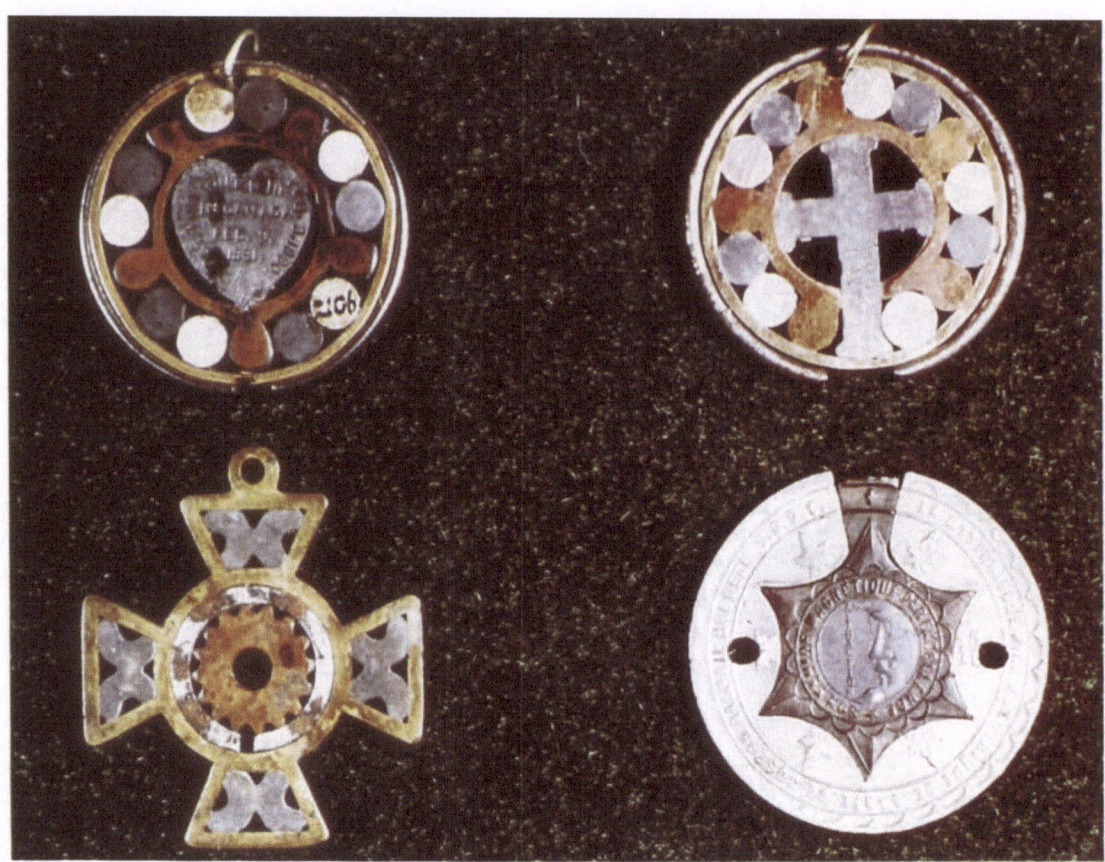

I

Modern electrogalvanic amulets for protection and cure of disease. The essential feature is the presence of two metals, generally copper and zinc and is an exploitation of the galvanic current of Galvani and Volta.

By courtesy of the Wellcome Trustees.

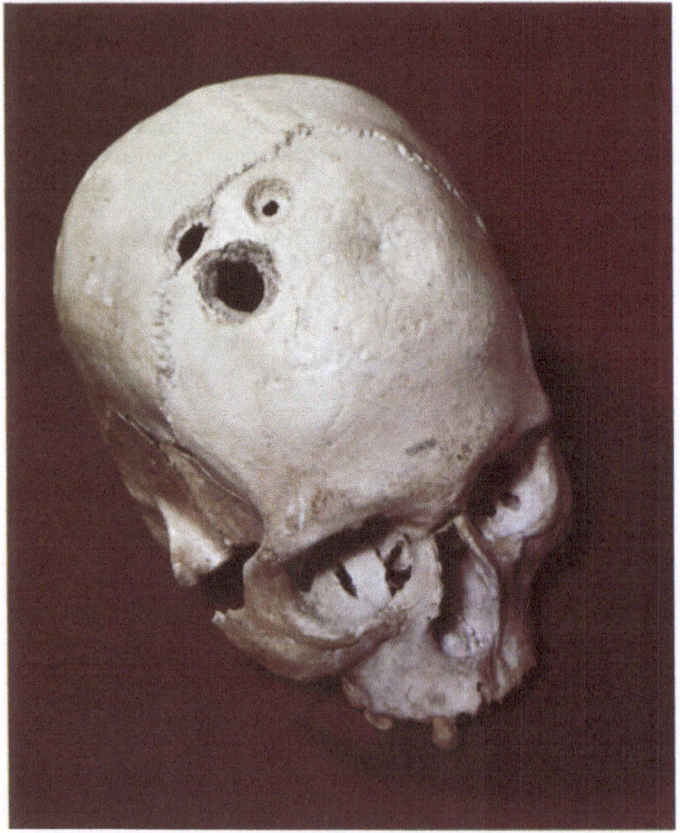

II

Trephined skull discovered by Dr Kathleen Kenyon's expedition to Jericho in January 1958. Found at a depth of about 12 feet in Tomb 88, a tomb cut in the rock. The cultural phase is intermediate between early and mid Bronze Age, circa 2200 BC.

By courtesy of the Wellcome Trustees.

history had to be taken in order to find out whether a taboo had been broken or an enemy offended, and then an examination made in his home for signs of a ritual that might have been used to invoke a spirit.

In the absence of a concept of disease entities, a history of the onset of symptoms and an examination for physical signs was unnecessary. Such a routine could not help towards finding a spiritual cause. The investigation necessary for this was a sort of a religious and legalistic enquiry, which required the general practitioner to combine the qualities of a priest, lawyer and detective rather than that of a physician. In the treatment he was required to be a sorcerer, and thus all-in-all had to be a man of considerable understanding of custom and belief, holding as a result a position of importance in the community. The object of diagnosis and treatment in such primitive communities is the discovery and removal of a cause, the nature of which is not physical. As such, it is the end of an evolutionary branch in the tree of medical history. It is not from these practitioners that the modern general medical practitioner springs.

THE DIAGNOSTIC SIGNIFICANCE OF DREAMS

Sigerist has set out the theory of disease aetiology and the development of ritual in diagnosis, treatment and prophylaxis, in the first volume of *Primitive and Archaic Medicine*, the history of medicine which he unfortunately did not live to complete. Some of these beliefs are particularly interesting as they have survived into later periods of practice and folk medicine.

There is a great deal of use of dreams in diagnosis and treatment. Dreams are a particularly vivid way of experiencing 'contact' with the dead, especially with the recent dead, and may be interpreted by the dreamer as visits from the spirits. In the Greek cult of Asklepios, sick people went to the temples to await in sleep the experience of a communion with the god and his healing power. This practice was known as incubation and not much of its detail has survived. The purpose of the priestly guardians of the temple seems to have been in the nature of selection of the patient, the dying being rigidly excluded. The process invoked was in the dreams of specific cures by the god, who was attended by his snakes. A late example of this cult may have taken place in the fourth century AD building, the ruins lying within the lines of an ancient hill fort on the right bank of the Severn at Lydney, near the beginnings of the Severn Bore. Here was a temple to Nodens, a god of hunting and of water. He had his counterpart in Nuadu of the Irish and Llud Llaw Eraint of the Welsh. Alongside the temple court is an open fronted building divided into cells, reminiscent of the type of structure in which the sick slept whilst awaiting the healing dreams. Nearby, there are baths and a guest house. The invocation of spirits in dreams and solicitation of their aid in causing or curing disease has analogies with modern sorcery.

EVIL SPIRITS

One of the primitive concepts of disease is known to anthropologists as 'the plus or minus theory', in which something is either added to or taken away from the body in order to cause the disturbance that gives rise to sickness. This could either be the removal of the occupying soul or the addition of an alien one, or the entry of such phenomena as 'elf shot', for which the Anglo-Saxons had magic formulae. Fetishes, which themselves may be possessed of a spirit, can be used either to cause or prevent disease, and the finding of them by modern 'witch doctors' in the investigation of a disease is of importance in the diagnosis. American Indians believed that medicine bundles possessed magical powers, and were often buried beneath the floors of their huts with the intention of either protecting or injuring the occupants.

The modern custom of wearing black for mourning has its roots in the ancient belief in evil spirits. People feared that ghosts of the recently dead might seek re-entry into living bodies and cause sickness. Near relatives were particularly vulnerable to this so they all dressed unusually by wearing black to make themselves unfamiliar to the spirit. Drawing the window curtains was also believed to discourage the spirit from re-entering the house. In more developed societies there were special demons of sickness which could bring illness.

Amulets, whose 'power' of prevention still command a sales value today (col. pl. I), are for prophylaxis only. The Neolithic practice of trepanation of the skull produced some early examples (col. pl. II). This operation was usually performed on the left of the skull, which suggests some sort of ritual significance (although it may also have been because righthanded men carried out the operations, facing their patients!). Bone healing points to the recovery of many of the subjects, even after multiple operations.

The operation, however, was also performed on the dead, which therefore suggests that the whole purpose of the operation was to obtain these *rondelles* of the skull. Many examples of these have survived, indicating that they were highly prized, possibly because they were used as amulets. Paul Broca (1824–1881), the pioneer neuro-surgeon, has written many papers on Neolithic trepanation.

3. Rowan tree loops used as protection against witches.
By courtesy of the Pitt Rivers Museum.

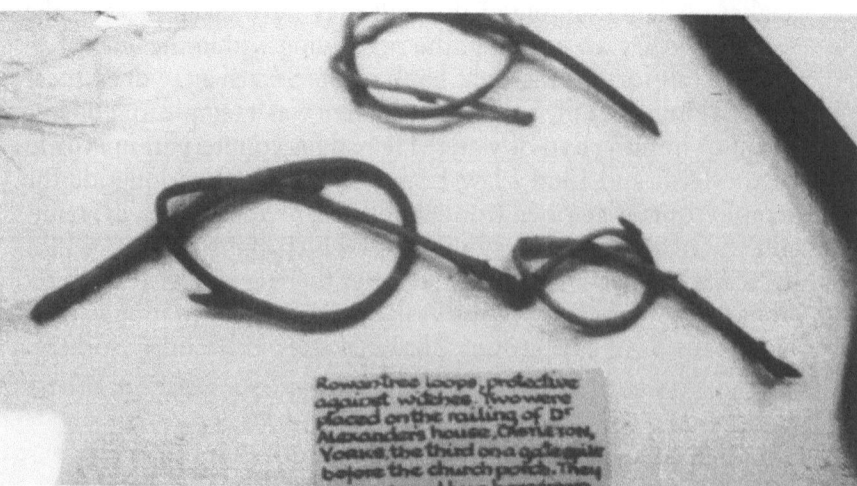

Amulets were used as charms against the powers of fetishes and of the evil eye to cause illness (figure 3). As it was impossible to distinguish who was possessed of these powers and from whence an attack could come, people used amulets for constant protection against all sources of evil, for unlike fetishes amulets only had the power to prevent illness. They were extremely popular in folk medicine and their use has continued into the twentieth century. In 1921, horse hair was found pegged to a door in Laugharne, Wales, to ward off the evil eye (col. pl. III).

The Druids

As early as the second century BC, the druids already had a reputation outside Gaul. Julius Caesar believed that the origins of druidism were to be found in Britain, and practitioners who would study the subject closely had to travel to Britain to do so. For their interest in medicine we have to rely on Pliny's *Natural History*, where he describes the ritual ceremony necessary for the collection of mistletoe, and its use 'taken in drink' to 'impart fecundity to barren animals' and as 'an antidote to all poisons'. The druidic association of the mistletoe with the oak is interesting in view of the rarity with which it is found on this tree in modern times. There were ritual instructions for the collection of *selago* (similar to savin, *Juniperus sabina*) the smoke of which was recommended in ophthalmic treatments. The marsh plant, *samolus* (brookweed, *S. valerandi*) if gathered 'with the left hand, when fasting' was used as a charm against diseases of cattle. The gatherer was enjoined not to look behind him, nor to lay the plant anywhere but in the drinking-troughs.

The whole subject of druidism has been bedevilled by anti-quarianism, but there is substantial evidence of a systematic organisation with educational, legal, political, religious and medico-magical functions. They are of particular interest for the early mention of the use of plants in treatment, though on a medico-magical, and not on a pharmacological, basis.

It is evident from Tacitus' account that the druids were still in Britain when they terrorised the Roman soldiery during Suetonius Paulinus' raid on Anglesey in AD 60. It is perhaps of significance that he does not mention them in the biography of his father-in-law Agricola, who administered Britain for seven years from AD 78. It may therefore be the story of the end of druidism, which it was the Roman policy to suppress. With the Roman soldiers came a new form of medicine.

The Roman Invasion of Britain

Julius Caesar first came to Britain in the year 55 BC, under-estimating the resistance both of the Channel and the inhabitants. He had to return in 54 BC with a better knowledge of the tides and a larger army before he could lay the foundations of the *Pax Romana*.

INFLUENCE ON BRITISH LIFE

The civilisation of the distant Roman Republic was far more advanced than anything this country had experienced: military and civil administration were of a scale that the natives had never contemplated. However, their interest in the invaders was aroused when they realised that their co-operation would bring them rewards in trade with Roman occupied Gaul. This commerce was mainly centred on the south eastern coast, where the advantages of friendly relations with the Roman merchants who followed in the wake of the army, were more immediately apparent.

Julius Caesar did not stay long as he was occupied with the Gallic Revolt and then the Civil Wars. However, the Roman influence remained for nearly 100 years after this military invasion, through the presence of the merchants. Initially they traded through the Channel route, but their influence gradually extended beyond the coastline. They familiarised the Britons with a new form of society and quietly prepared the way for the government that was to come later.

The lack of political agreement amongst the many native tribes often resulted in an unsettled leadership and jealous contestants for power. Some factions solicited Roman support and their rulers adopted titles such as *rex*, but this implied Roman recognition rather than Romanisation. Little is known of their social structure and we can only learn about their medical practice from the Roman accounts of the druids and our own surmises of the nature of early medicine. At this stage there is no evidence that the Romans who came and went had any organised medical service in Britain. The traditional household remedies, beloved of the Roman *paterfamilias*, would have provided some comfort for the Roman merchants.

ANTI-ROMAN FEELING

It was inevitable that some anti-Roman feeling would grow amongst those who felt they had a grievance against the foreigners. By AD 40, the unrest had reached proportions which seemed to threaten the Continent, albeit remotely. The Romans were faced with the choice of either creating an Atlantic Frontier on the bounds of the Empire, or of conquering and garrisoning Britain; roughly the same number of men would have been required for either. The Roman expansionist policy favoured the advantages of a garrison that could be paid for out of a new territory, exploited for fresh revenue. It was better than using an equally costly force within the old boundaries, at a charge to the existing budget. For these and other reasons in AD 43, Claudius, accompanied by the Second Augusta, the Ninth Hispana, the Fourteenth Gemina and the Twentieth Valeria Victrix Legions, invaded and began the conquest of the island.

The Development of Roman Medical Practice

The legions brought with them a new sort of medicine adapted to the practical requirements of an army in the field. However, in Rome itself, the citizens had never given much of their time to theorising and such scientific medicine as they possessed was directly due to Greek influence. The Augustan Roman country landowner saw himself as a lover of nature, who looked after his *familia rustica* with good old-fashioned remedies. Their own tradition, dating from long before the second Punic War of about 214 BC, had been of a primitive nature, characterised by specialist deities and their dedicated temples. The Etruscans and other early Italians had also left a religious legacy.

THE IMPORTANCE OF GREEK MEDICINE

To understand Roman medical practice, it is necessary to go back to Greek medicine. The Greek concept of medicine, combining scientific enquiry and applied theory, and the belief in searching out knowledge for its own sake, laid the foundations of rational medicine. The history of the Greeks from Magna Grecia through the Ionian and Athenian to the Alexandrian Schools is illuminated by such names as Pythagoras, Empedocles, Hippocrates, Plato, Aristotle, Erasistratus and Herophilus. It is a story of expanding knowledge, bringing escape from the older, primitive notions of disease.

Asclepiades of Bithynia in Asia Minor, is generally considered to be the man who introduced Greek medicine to Rome. In the last century BC he brought to Rome the idea of a solidist theory to replace the humoral theory of the Hippocratic School. In its simplest terms this postulated that the body was made up of an infinite number of atoms, the mechanical movements of which constituted life. His pupil, Themison of Laodicea, developed his theory that combinations of atoms formed tubular spaces called pores, into the appealingly simple doctrine of the Methodists. Disease depended on whether the pores were open or closed, *status strictus* or *status laxus* and treatment was directed to correcting an abnormal excess. There was also, conveniently, a *status mixtus* which allowed for a certain nicety in diagnosis. This system became popular in Caesar's Rome and was associated with Epicureanism.

In the first century AD, the Pneumatists, who were associated with the Stoicism which so appealed to the stern disciplined Roman, developed the complex pulse lore. The quality of the pulse revealed the state of the *Pneuma* or Vital Air, on which they believed the life force depended. Later Pneumatists, who preferred to call themselves Eclectics, revived the humoral theories of Hippocrates and felt the need to combat *dyscrasia*.

INFLUENCE OF GREEK MEDICINE IN ROME

The arrival of Greek hostages in Rome introduced the Greek idea of medicine. However, the general scientific principles of the Greeks were seldom understood even by educated Romans. The possibility that the cause of illness was to be found in disturbances within the body due to physical causes with direct physical remedies such as diet, exercise, drugs, massage, plasters and baths appealed to the Roman's preference for straightforwardness.

The temptation grew to apply 'proven' remedies in a stereotyped manner, with perhaps the occasional backward glance to the magic of the *haruspex*, the ancient Roman soothsayer and reader of entrails, who was of Etruscan origin.

The Work of Celsus

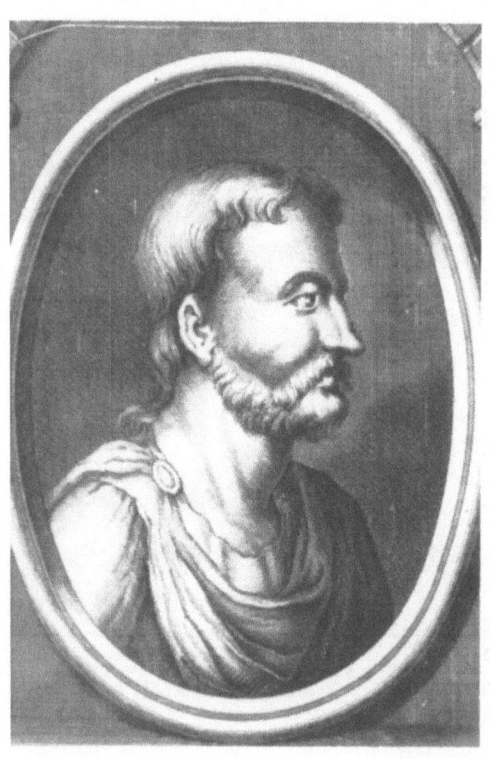

1. A.Cornelius Celsus. Engraving by J. Spyck, in the Wellcome Institute. *By courtesy of the Wellcome Trustees.*

The *De Medicina* written by Celsus (figure 1) in about AD 30, is the earliest known medical work in Latin. The material for this, however, was almost certainly Greek in origin and largely of the Alexandrian School. His treatise is composed of eight books dealing with medical history, diet, hygiene, therapeutics including drugs and physiotherapy, pathology, internal and external diseases and surgery; there is a special passage on military surgery. It is a scientific work, recognising the importance of anatomy as a basis for the study of medicine, and stressing the need for diagnosis before treatment.

In this work, Celsus emphasises the role of physical science in place of the spiritual magic of the primitives. He writes of popular magic almost apologetically, but nevertheless, with the reservation that there might just be something in it. The practical treatment of quinsy includes fomentations, gargles, local applications and surgical incision. However, he concludes with a reference to the speculative use of a nestling swallow, burned, preserved in salt and crumbled into ash to be taken with hydromel as a draught. He then adds the disclaimer, 'Since this remedy has considerable popular authority, and cannot possibly be a danger although I have not read of it in medical authorities, yet I thought it should be inserted here in my work'. Some ideas of sympathetic magic also intrude, with such remedies as worms boiled in oil for treatment of maggots in the ear, but he does not give them prominence.

Celsus carefully notes physical signs. A particularly good

example of this is his instruction for taking the pulse:

. . . the bath and exercise and fear and anger and any other feeling of the mind is often apt to excite the pulse; so that when the practitioner makes his first visit, the solicitude of the patient who is in doubt as to what the practitioner may think of his state, may disturb his pulse. On this account a practitioner of experience does not seize the patient's forearm with his hand, as soon as he comes, but first sits down and with a cheerful countenance asks how the patient finds himself; and if the patient has any fear, he calms him with entertaining talk, and only after that moves his hand to touch the patient.

His description of the four classical signs of inflammation is even more well known:

Notae vero inflammationis sunt quattuor:
rubor et tumor cum calore et dolore.

He describes the extraction of missiles, the treatment of fractures by reduction and splinting, and the use of the trephine for depressed fractures of the skull. His notes on surgery include catheterisation, cutting for stone, excision of nasal polyps, paracentesis abdominis, operations for hernia, hydrocoele and fistulae, and stress the importance of skin and muscle flaps in amputation. He recommends many external applications including saline, essential oils, pitch and turpentine for wounds. Internally, it is chiefly clysters, purgatives, vomits, anodynes and antidotes that comprise the pharmacopoeia.

THE EMPIRIC SCHOOL

In the historical account given in his *Prooemium* to *De Medicina*, Celsus writes favourably of the Empiric School, whose practical outlook would naturally appeal to the Roman. Its followers relied on experience rather than on theory, adopting the motto, 'Diseases are cured not by argument but by medicine'. It began in the third century BC as a reaction against the theorising of the Dogmatic or Rationalist School founded on the Hippocratic Corpus. Symptoms and symptom complexes were studied in preference to disease theories and attention was given particularly to symptomatic relief. Whilst this is of great clinical significance it has many limitations restricting the advance of knowledge, but its appeal has continued to attract orthodox doctors and 'fringe practitioners' up to the present day.

Medical Care in the Army

At the end of his historical account, Celsus states that he is 'of the opinion that the Art of Medicine ought to be rational, but to draw instruction from evident causes, all obscure ones being rejected from the practice of the Art, although not from the practitioner's study'. This 'useful' knowledge was applied with typical Roman thoroughness and organisation to the provision of a military medical service. Julius Caesar encouraged Greek doctors to live in Rome when, in 46 BC, he 'conferred citizenship on all practitioners of medicine and all professors of liberal arts in Rome, to make them more desirous of living in the city and to induce others to come there'. It has been suggested that this was in fact a diplomatic move really intended to create a Roman military medical service.

There were skilled practitioners with the army, for it is known that Scribonius Largus of the Empiric School accompanied Claudius on the expedition to Britain. He dedicated his work *Compositiones Medicamentorum* to the Emperor, in which he describes the process of extracting opium from the poppy by slitting the capsule, allowing the extruded juice to dry *in situ*, then scraping it off and rolling it into a ball. This manoeuvre, unlike many subsequent descriptions of the use of the poppy, succeeded in obtaining the active constituent. Dioscorides, a slightly later and more eminent pioneer pharmacologist, did not come to Britain, but was a military surgeon in Nero's army. It was during this service that he gathered together much of his botanical information. These two distinguished medical men, however, may not have been typical of the serving medical officer for they were probably in the nature of personal attendants.

ORGANISATION OF MEDICAL STAFF IN THE ROMAN ARMY

The Roman generals were well aware of the importance to morale that care for the wounded soldier provided, and at the time of Caesar's edict in 46 BC, the wounded were already being evacuated from the field by wagon. The rank and file had their own practitioners, although the nature of their organisation and training is not altogether clear. References in Cicero and Celsus suggest that some were educated, and Augustus granted the equestrian dignity *dignitas equestrias* with the right to wear the ring of the knightly class, to all free physicians including educated army surgeons.

It would appear that by the time of Trajan and Hadrian (AD 98–138) there was an established military medical service. Trajan's column shows the army dressers, *capsarii* (their name is derived from the round box *capsa*, in which they carried the bandages), bandaging the legionaries. Their medical counterparts were the ranker orderlies, *medici ordinarii*. Both the *capsarii* and the *medici ordinarii* were non-combatant. A legion of between 5,000 to 7,000 men had a legionary medical officer, *medicus legionis* and each of the legion's ten cohorts had four cohort medical officers, *medici cohortis*. The medical staff ranked in status with the NCOs, *principales*, and other civilian bureaucrats attached to the army who were without internal rank structure. The army also had its own wound surgeons, *medici vulnerarii*, and wounds were bandaged from the earliest days of the citizen army. Malingerers had even been known to use bandages in order to feign injury so that they could avoid service under the unpopular Appius Claudius about 469 BC! Members of the medical staff were all directly responsible to the *praefectus castrorum*. This officer, third in line of command in the camp, was usually a professional soldier promoted from amongst the senior centurions.

ROMAN MILITARY HOSPITALS

The design of the legionary hospitals, *valetudinaria*, provides a striking example of the efficiency of the Roman army medical service and its high standard of medical care (figure 2). Each of the hospitals was under the command of an *optio valetudinarius*. There are remains of these hospitals in Britain at Inchtuthill and Caerleon, and smaller ones are at Housesteads, Fendoch, Birrens and Pen Llystyn.

The general plan is reminiscent of the tented Roman military hospital. It has a central courtyard around which there is a rectangular corridor. On three sides of the courtyard, the corridor is lined by an inner and outer row of small wards; these are usually grouped in pairs, opening onto the corridor through a small vestibule which gives access to a latrine for each pair.

The outer wards at Caerleon are in groups of three. The archaeologists, however, have not discovered any latrines and provision for heating is apparent in only one room. There was obviously

:. Reconstruction of the valetudinarium at Vetera. After R Schultze: photo Rheinisches Landesmuseum, Bonn.

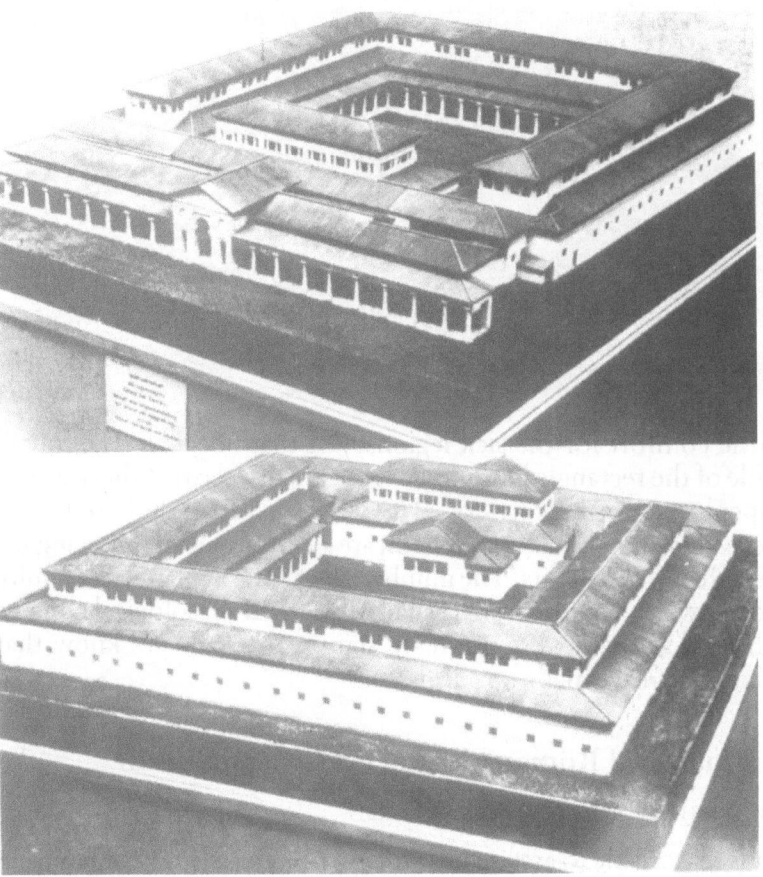

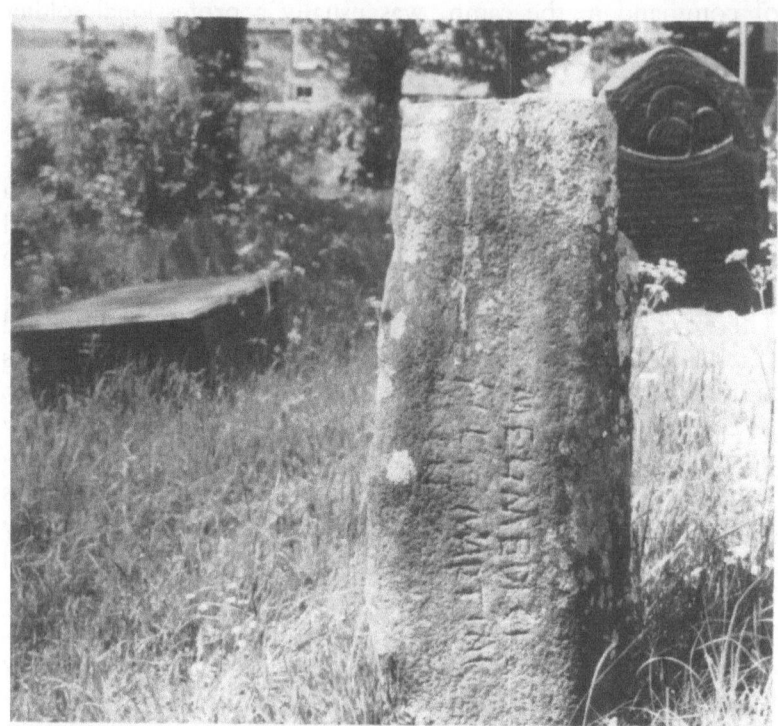

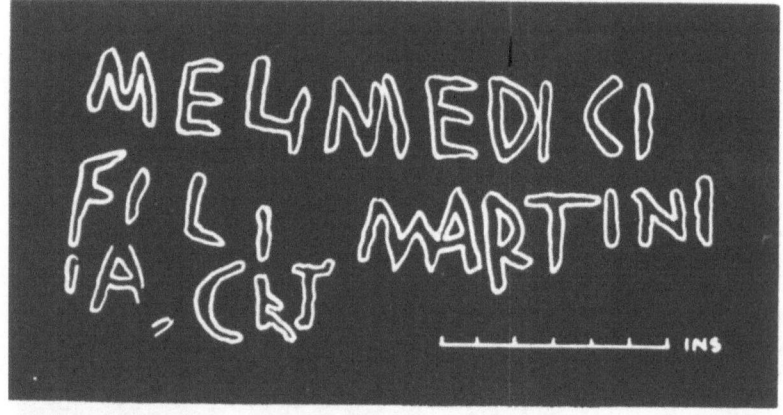

3. An ancient inscribed stone in the churchyard at Llangîan, Caernarvonshire.
Crown copyright. Reproduced by permission of Her Majesty's Stationery Office and the Royal Commission on Ancient and Historical Monuments in Wales.

4. A tracing of the inscription on the stone shown in figure 3. The inscription reads, 'MELI MEDICI FILI MARTINI IACIT'.

little comfort for the sick legionary at that hospital. The fourth side of the rectangle is occupied by a casualty clearing theatre, also opening onto the corridor. The wards at Inchtuthill are fifteen feet square and those at Caerleon are slightly smaller, allowing for less than five patients. The number of wards was planned carefully to allow for a five per cent casualty list: the archaeological remains show that there were normally sixty wards, and we know that sixty *centuriae* made up a legion.

Influence of Roman Medical Practice on Britain

BRITISH RECRUITMENT IN THE ARMY

It is reasonable to assume that the type of knowledge contained in Celsus's *De Medicina* was available to the Roman legions in

Britain and, with increasing Romanisation of the countryside, to the Briton as well. As the occupation of Britain was consolidated, conscription and recruitment to the Roman Army took place from amongst the native inhabitants which was in accordance with the general policy of the Empire. The medical service enlisted freedmen or foreigners as *medici ordinarii* for the auxiliary troops and the British auxiliary regiments, recruited under Trajan, played a gallant part in his campaigns. The medical organisation for the irregular formations of cavalry and infantry, known as *cunei*, *vexillationes* and *numeri*, remains even more obscure than it does for the auxiliary troops.

Aurelian (AD 270–275) stated that there should be 'free medical treatment for the soldier' (*milites a medicis gratis currentur*). If this aphorism held any truth, the British recruit must have had some practical experience of medical care, and would have had the opportunity of becoming familiar with Roman medicine.

The name of one of the medical orderlies has survived in the memorial to the *medicus ordinarius* at Housesteads, on the Roman Wall: Anicius Ingenuus of the First Cohort of the Tungrians was only 25 when he died in about the year AD 83. The first named British medical practitioner is on the fifth to early sixth century tombstone, now in the parish churchyard of Llangîan in Llŷn (figure 3). In style and form this is Celtic. Alcock affirms this from the vertical inscription in the manner of the Ogam script, and by the name alone of the deceased appearing in the genitive case. This distinguished the Welsh memorials from those of the continentals. Nothing is known of this Melus the son of Martin, other than the words inscribed on the stone (figure 4). In the word *medicus*, however, there is evidence of Roman influence. The word later passed into Welsh as *meddyg*.

ROMANISATION OF BRITAIN

Whereas the Romans took great care to leave native customs and practices undisturbed when they did not interfere with government, many Britons voluntarily adopted Roman ways. Settled landowners copied Roman villas within a generation of the conquest; later on even bath houses were added, a feature which had not been particularly popular at first! As the towns grew, British craftsmen and traders joined the Roman inhabitants and Roman standards of hygiene became accepted in the urban settlements. Although there is no firm evidence of the nature of civilian medical practice, it seems probable that some Roman treatment, even if only that given by a retired *medicus*, who had remained after his army service, would occasionally have been accepted. Gradually, Roman citizenship was extended and in AD 213 this privilege was given to all freeborn provincials.

3
The
Anglo-Saxons
and Celts

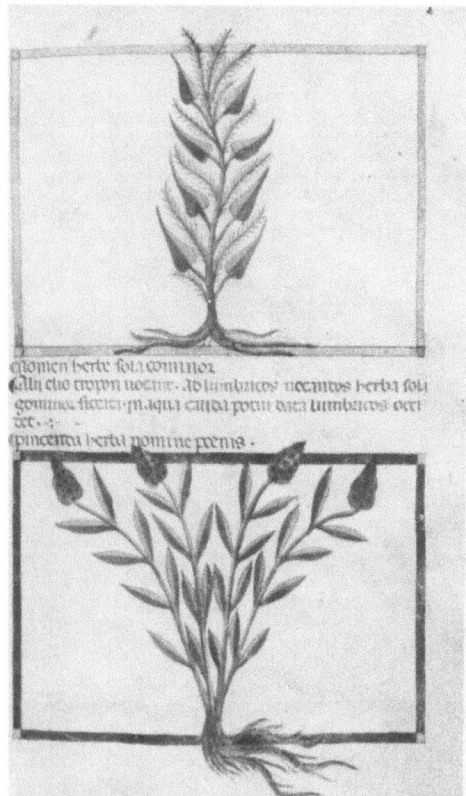

Anglo-Saxon Invasions of Britain

Military disasters in the Empire during the fifth century AD loosened the Roman hold on Britain and consequently left its citizens prey to attacks across the old frontiers by the Picts from Scotland and the Scots from Northern Ireland. The Saxons from Germany had carried on a legitimate trade as well as intermittent raids on the island. They saw in the dissolution of the existing Roman power an opportunity for conquest. Joined by their neighbours the Angles, Frisians and possibly the Jutes, they had established themselves in Britain as Anglo-Saxons by AD 600.

Trevelyan, the Cambridge historian, thought that the Romans left behind them only three permanent legacies, 'the traditional site of London, the Roman roads and Welsh Christianity'. Their Anglo-Saxon successors were barbarians who did not bring any scientific learning and contributed nothing to the Roman store of medical knowledge. The only lore they possessed was based on the healing rites of a pagan religious medicine, some primitive knowledge of herbs and the rough and ready first aid of the pirate.

Medical Practice In The Church

Christianity had been the official religion in the Roman Empire for a hundred years before the legions left Britain. However, its practice had largely disappeared before the arrival of Augustine in AD 567, except in the Celtic Churches of Wales and Ireland. This picture was changed with the advent of the Christian mission.

MEDICAL EDUCATION – THE ROLE OF THE CHURCH

Improvement in the medical field came with the arrival of the new Christians. When Theodore the Greek had been appointed Archbishop of Canterbury, one of his first acts was to found a school at Canterbury, where all the liberal arts could be studied. Dr Charles Talbot, the eminent medievalist and medical historian, states that medicine was included in the curriculum because 'St Aldhelm, a pupil there, mentioned it as one of the subjects studied alongside astronomy and arithmetic'. He also notes that St John of Beverley, criticising the action of a physician, said, 'I remember that Archbishop Theodore . . . used to say it was dangerous to bleed at a time when the light of the moon and the pull of the tides was increasing'.

Although it is not known which texts were studied, the emphasis would have been on Greek medical philosophy. These medical advances, however, were mostly lost in the ensuing centuries of Danish invasion when the libraries were destroyed and the monasteries pillaged.

TEXTS STUDIED BY BEDE

It is not known which texts were available for study, although the possibilities are discussed in Talbot's *Medicine in Medieval England*. Bede (AD 673–735) had an incomplete copy of Pliny's *Historia Naturalis* and he had access to a book on regimen which Paul of Aegina attributed to Diocles of Carystus, a Greek eclectic of the fourth century BC. He also had a good copy of the Latin work of Cassius Felix on Greek Medicine (AD 447), a compilation from Soranus and Galen, for he quotes the whole chapter on dysentery in his own *Retractions*.

HERBALS

Botanical herbals were of the greatest importance in early medical treatments. Bishop Cynehard of Winchester wrote to Mainz for medical books as those already in his library gave only foreign medicinal plants. The herbals could have been copies of the Dioscorides manuscripts made in about AD 512 for Juliana Anicia, and are known as the Codex Juliana Anicia (*Codex Vindobonensis*). He may also have had the manuscript herbal of Pseudo-Apuleius, originally compiled about AD 400 from Greek material (figure 1). The author is known as Pseudo-Apuleius to distinguish him from the author of the *Golden Ass*. The earliest known copy of this herbal dates from the seventh century AD and is now kept at Leiden.

Drawings in successive herbal manuscripts that had been copied from each other and not from nature, were debased to figures bearing little resemblance to the plants in the description (col. pl. IV). These herbals were of foreign origin and foreign nomenclature. The Bishop of Winchester was hoping to acquire a text that would help him to identify native species with similar properties to foreign plants, a task that was virtually impossible with the illustrations from some of the copies.

PRACTICAL APPLICATION OF MEDICAL KNOWLEDGE

The Church believed it had a Christian duty to care for the sick and did so in its own enclosed communities. In the Rule of St Benedict, first formulated in about AD 516, there are specific instructions for looking after sick monks in Anglo-Saxon monasteries. The Church also carried out healing functions, similar to those of the pagan deities, with miraculous cures attributed to the saints and holy relics. Bede's *Ecclesiastical History* gives many examples.

The cure of disease, and often its cause, was accepted as a spiritual rather than physical process. In particular, there is the ritual for casting out demons by exorcists. Success here depended upon the degree of suggestibility in the sufferer and the power of the priest to manipulate it (col. pl. V).

DEVELOPMENT OF HOSPITALS

It was natural that the theoretical interest in the classical medical works shown by the early English Churchmen should be put to practical use. In such communities, as well as the Christian duty of mercy there was the practical duty of care for those in their own enclosed community who became old, sick or infirm. By an extension of the disciplined care given, such institutions later provided a similar service for the people. There is evidence showing the existence of both clerical and non-clerical practitioners in Anglo-Saxon England and in Wales with both clerical and non-clerical hospitals in England. It is pointless to distinguish the function of such a *laēce hus, hospitium* or infirmary from a place to provide shelter and care.

A plan exists for the construction of a separate medical unit in the Irish monastery of St Gall in Switzerland. It incorporates a pharmacy, herb garden, wards for the seriously ill, recovery rooms after blood letting, bathrooms and lavatories. Unfortunately, it is not known whether or not this was ever built.

Bede had written of the laundry arrangements in the hospitals of his time, when Bethwegen washed mantles and garments for use there. He also referred to a house where 'those that were ill and likely to die shortly' were carried, as was Caedmon in about AD 680. A hospital, St Peter's at York, was said to have been founded by King Athelstan about 937 on the site of the present Theatre Royal. There were two tenth century Anglo-Saxon hospitals at Worcester which, like that at York, seem to have been extra-mural to the monasteries.

Medical Practice Outside The Church

The popular conception of the Anglo-Saxon leech has its origins in the documents of a much later date than those of Bede. The leech books are the result of the movement toward a nationalist scholarship, inspired by Alfred the Great who encouraged the translation of Latin works into English. *Lāece* is the Anglo-Saxon word for physician, and the medieval word became *leche*. The earliest leech book to survive is that of Bald and is believed to have been written in the second half of the tenth century, but is itself a copy of an earlier version. It is based on the work of the Greek Alexandrian School, and in particular on Galen, that had been compiled and translated into Latin by Oribasius and Paul of Aegina. The later Anglo-Saxon text, the *Peri Didaxeon*, is a partial translation of Petrocellus, whose writings are also to be found in the Leech Book of Bald. These works do not represent the folk medicine of the barbarous Anglo-Saxon pirates, but are in the tradition of the Greek School (col. pl. VI).

The later, more complex, work called *Lacnunga* (the name comes from the Anglo-Saxon word *lāecung* which means healing), is based on remedies and magic derived from the classical world, and Celtic and Teutonic sources. It is a compilation of the medical lore that was available in Anglo-Saxon England, but it does not give an overall view of the medical and scientific beliefs of the time, unlike the monk Byrhtferth's *Manual* which deals with elementary science in astronomy, mathematics and the calendar.

Anglo-Saxon translations of herbals were also available to the practitioner. The Anglo-Saxon herbal contained in *Cotton Vitellius* MS CIII made in about 950, describes 132 plants from the *Herbarium* of Apuleius and 33 from Dioscorides. The *Codex Hertensis 192*, of ninth century English origin, includes the work of Dioscorides, Antonius Musa and Sextus Placitus (col. pl. VII).

POPULAR BELIEFS AND REMEDIES

In the realms of magic, people believed that diseases in man and animals could be caused by elf shot, that is, arrows shot by elves, for which flint arrow heads were often later mistaken. The only physical signs sought were those of skin puncture or denting. They were treated with charms and incantations, and talismans were used for prophylaxis. The 'white stone' was particularly recommended by the leech books to ward off elf shot, and it also included protection against flying venoms, aesir shot (from the gods) hag shot (from witches), and generally guarded against *brōc*, all unknown maladies. These magic rites against elves gradually became confused with the religious rites against demons.

SURGERY

Surgical procedures included incision (surgeon's knife, *lāece-seax*) blood letting (vein knife, *aedre-seax*) and cautery with the hot iron. Cupping was also practised with glass or horn. The Anglo-Saxon story of St Ethelrida suggests that physicians practised surgery. The physician (*lāece*) Cynifrid was called to open the chronic swelling beneath St Ethelrida's jaw; although he let the noxious matter out she died three days later. Cynifrid was probably a non-clerical practitioner of the Isle of Ely.

Blood letting was an attempt to correct any imbalance of the humours, which caused disease, or simply to let out an evil humour. Certain days, known as *Dies Aegytiaci* after the fourth century AD, were considered unfavourable for blood letting. In the Middle Ages blood letting diagrams were marked with the signs of the zodiac and a definite astrological relationship emerged.

Fractures were treated by bandages, to immobilise the limbs, as in the case of the unfortunate Bothelm, who slipped from a pinnacle during the building of Hexham Priory in the time of

Bishop Wilfrid, and broke both his arms and his legs. The Leech Book advised a splint after protecting the limb with a salve and elm-rind, renewing the treatment until the limb was healed. If it became gangrenous, an amputation was to be carried out through healthy tissue. Wounds were sewn with silk thread after injury and after deliberate surgery, such as that practised on hare lip.

Medical Laws Determining Physicians' Fees

THE LAW OF COMPENSATION

The early laws of compensation, including the *Leis Willelme* of William the Conquerer, were designed to control the vengeance of relatives. They determined that in feuds, murders and acts of revenge, the injured party should receive compensation from the injurer. The development of these laws passed through many stages: from mutilation of the assailant, through payment in kind, to compensation entirely in the form of money. This led to the development of the physician's fee.

IRISH LAW OF COMPENSATION: *Folog Nothrusa*

In early Irish Law, the expenses of the injured had to be met, wholly or partly, by the injurer until his victim was well again. In the Irish obligation of *othrus*, the duty of meeting the costs of all the necessities of treatment and maintenance fell upon the assailant. If the patient was treated in his own home instead of being maintained and treated elsewhere at the expense of the injurer, he was supplied with 'food and leech'. This later development was known as *tincisin*.

WELSH LAW OF COMPENSATION

It may have been that some medical treatment in Wales was free, but the laws show that in certain cases the physician was permitted to charge for treatment given outside the court and royal household, and he was entitled to payment in cases governed by the law of compensation.

The Welsh laws actually state the amount payable to the mediciner 'by the person who had wounded the patient':

For each of the three mortal wounds (namely a blow on the head unto the brain, a blow on the body unto the bowels, and the breaking of one of the four limbs) the mediciner should be given nine score pence and his food; or a pound without his food. He is to have twenty-four pence for applying a tent.

(The word 'tent' was used in late Middle English for a roll of absorbent material to keep a wound open.) He was to have twelve pence for treating a major blood vessel and eight pence for a

IV
(Above) The serpent whose bite is cured by the plant Viperina;
(Below) A very degraded copy of a drawing of the plant Acorus. Both from the Pseudo-Apuleius herbal in Wellcome MS 573.
By courtesy of the Wellcome Trustees.

V
St Benedict casting out devils from a possessed monk. Mural by Sodoma. Photograph by author.
Murals at the Abbey of Monte Olivetto Maggiore.

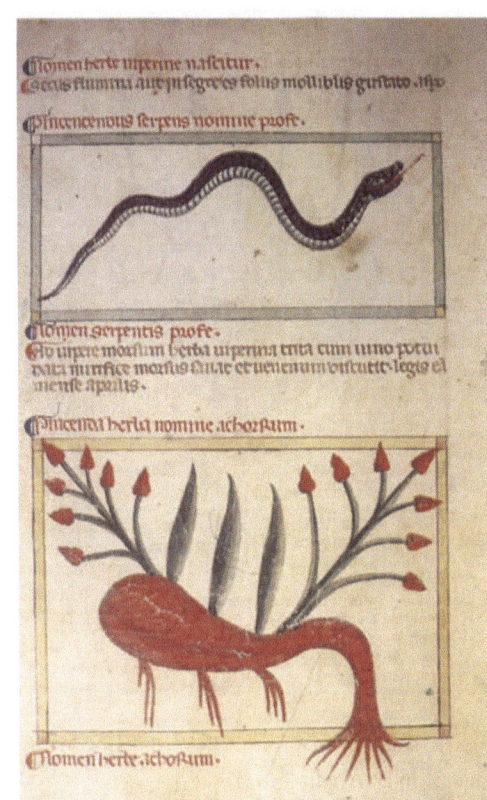

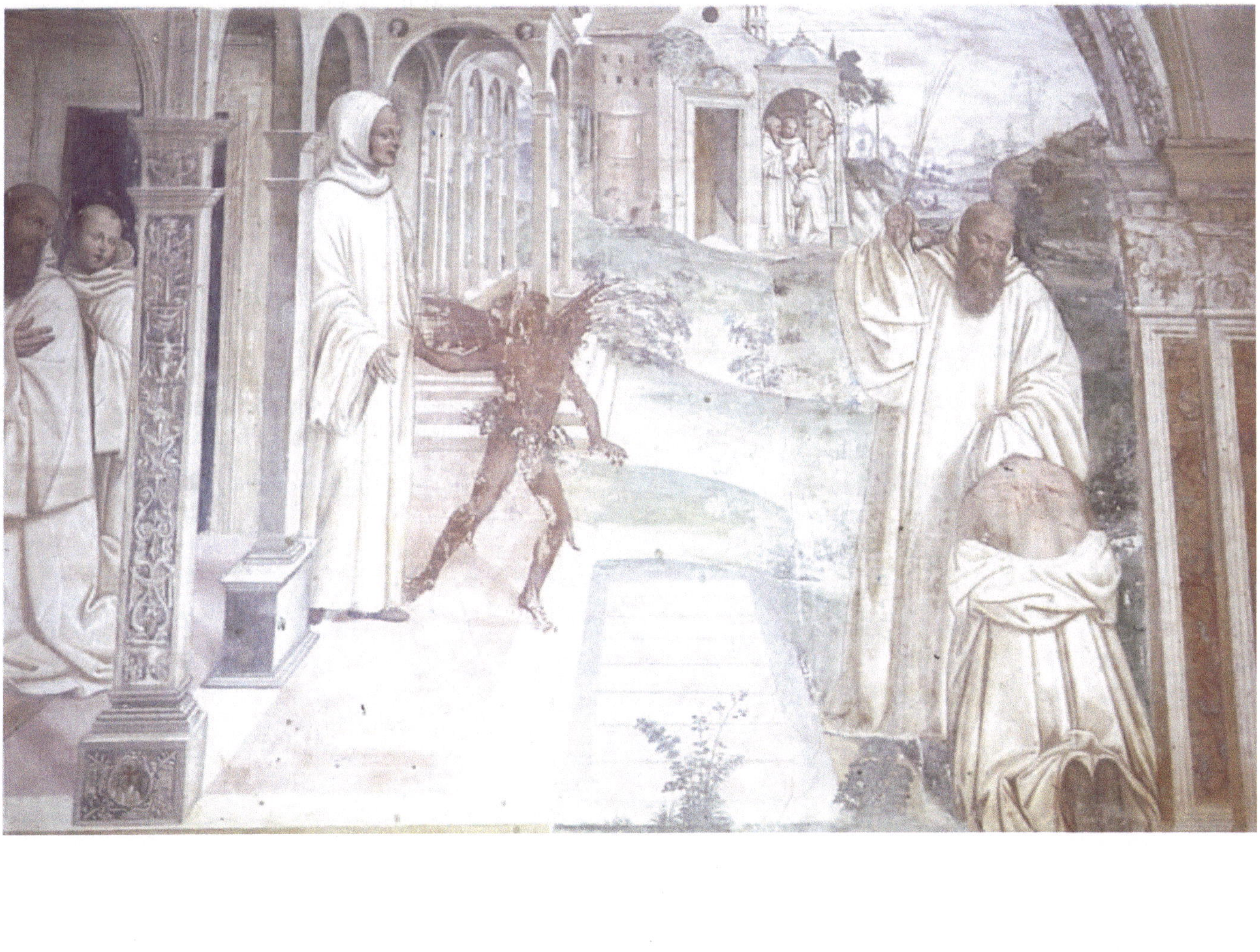

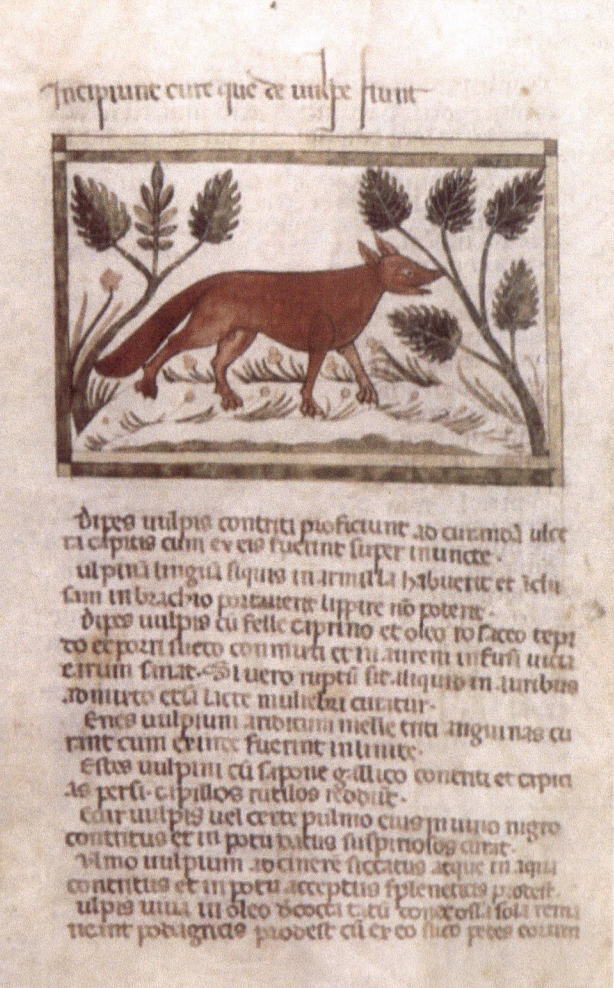

VI
A page from an Anglo-Saxon
medical recipe book, Wellcome MS 46.
From the original fragment in
the Wellcome Library. It includes
recipes for heartache, lung disease,
tumours and liver disease.
'For liver disease, take liverwort; let
it be carried home under your knee;
boil it in milk from a cow of one
colour and mix butter with it'.
By courtesy of the Wellcome Trustees.

VII
Animal remedies were used in
Anglo-Saxon England and this
illustration of the fox is taken from a
later copy of Sextus Placitus'
Medicina de Quadrupedibus found
in the mid thirteenth century.
Wellcome MS 573.
By courtesy of the Wellcome Trustees.

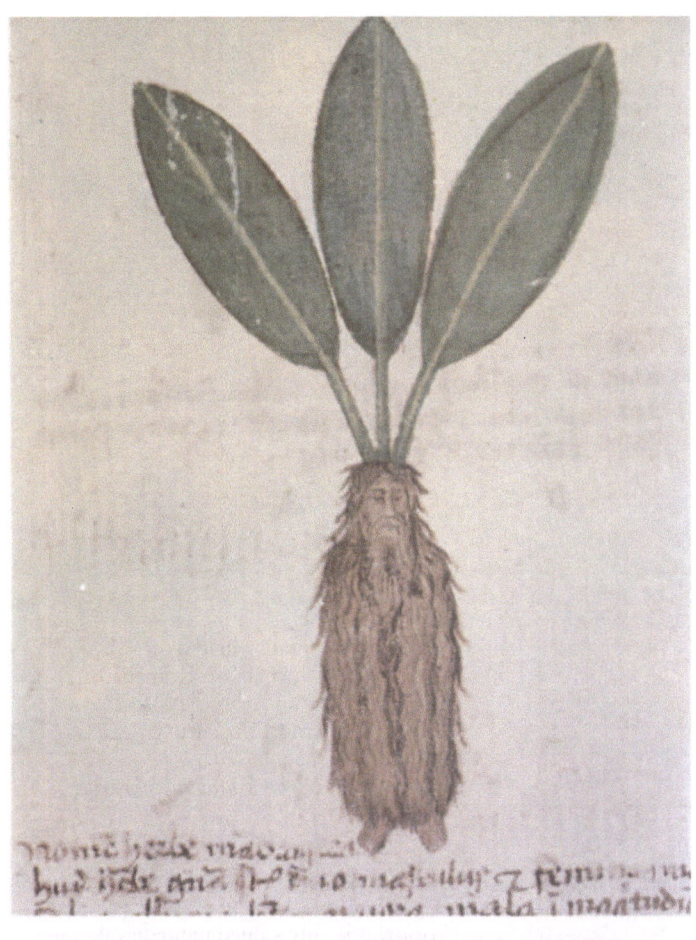

X
The root of the mandrake (*Atropa mandragora*), used as an aphrodisiac, was said to have been known to the Egyptians as 'Phallus of the Field' and to the Arabs as 'Devils' Testicles'. It was also taken in wine as a soporific. From the mid fifteenth century *Pseudo-Apuleius Herbarium* in Wellcome MS 574. *By courtesy of the Wellcome Trustees.*

XI
The mandrake root was removed by a dog. From the mid thirteenth century *Pseudo-Apuleius Herbarium* in Wellcome MS 573. *By courtesy of the Wellcome Trustees.*

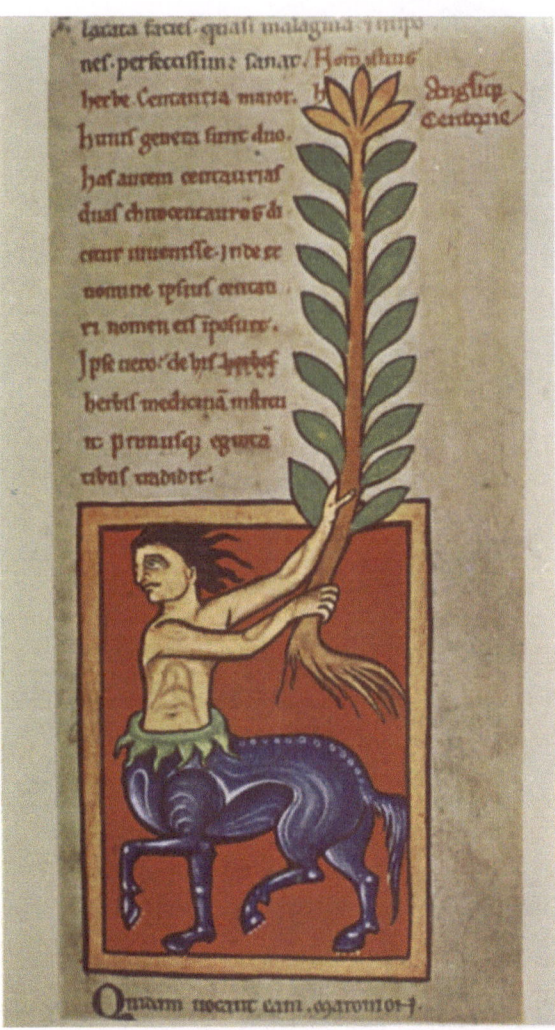

VIII
The plant Centaury held by a Centaur. A Norman or 'Romanesque' illustration from Ashmole MS 1462 folio 23, a thirteenth century Anglo-Norman herbal.
By courtesy of the Bodleian Library.

IX
The Mandrake. The mandrake root was highly valued in medieval medicine. It was said to resemble a human body in shape. Modern name: *Mandragora officinalis*. *Photograph by Robin Price, in the Chelsea Physic Garden.*

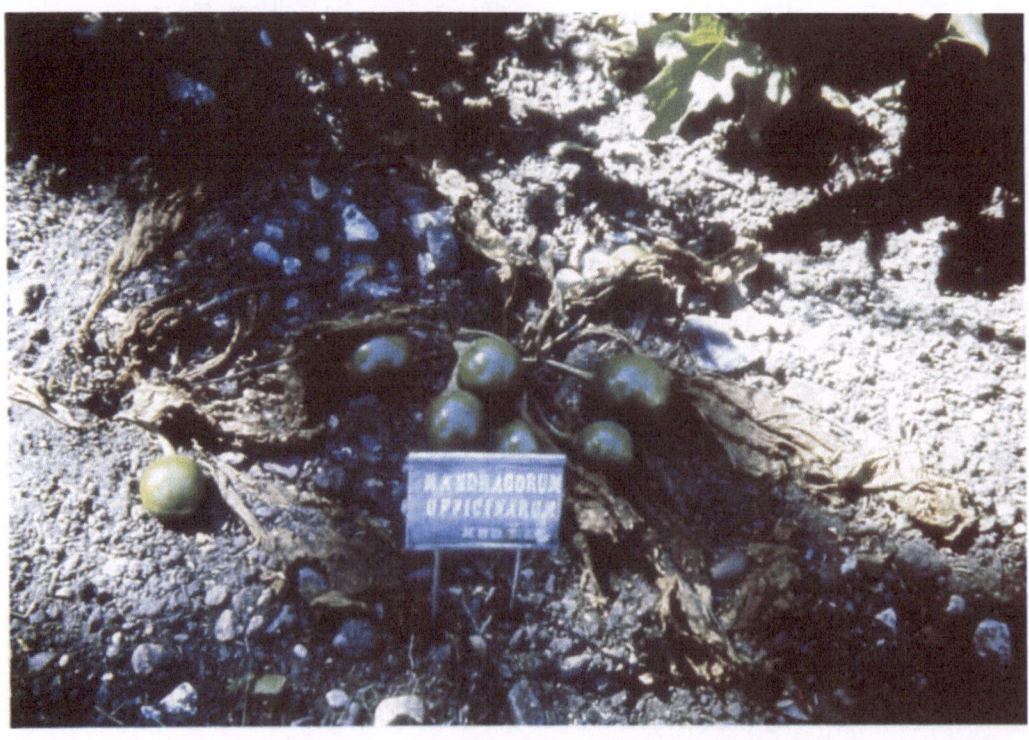

medicament of herbs to apply to a swelling. The Welsh laws also assess the amount of compensation payable to the victim in cases where medical treatment was not necessary, such as loss of hair from hair-pulling in anger.

If the mediciner was supplied with food, his fee was correspondingly diminished. The thirteenth century manuscript (Physicians of Myddfai) states that a fee of one pound without victuals, or nine score pence with victuals should be paid for treating a head wound exposing the brain. The charge for keeping the mediciner was probably one penny halfpenny for his 'nightly food', (the custom was to have two meals a day and nightly food refers to the passage of time rather than a specific meal) and a penny for his light. Records suggest that a bill of 60 pence could be presented to the assailant for the upkeep of the mediciner attending a patient with a mortal wound. At a rate of one halfpenny a day, the expected duration of medical attendance was 40 days.

The fees for specific treatment seem generous in comparison with the subsistence allowance, but they should also be compared with the fees charged for other services and the actual purchasing power of the money. The Welsh laws state that a judge received 24 pence for each judge examined for appointment. They also establish that a palfrey was worth six score pence, a working horse three score pence, a salmon net twenty-four pence, and a salmon two pence. A lamb was worth one penny and a sheep four pence, but a kitten with unopened eyes and a mouse-killing cat, ranked equally with a new-born lamb and a sheep.

DETAILS OF MEDICAL PRACTICE ILLUSTRATED IN IRISH AND WELSH LAWS

The early Welsh and Irish laws provide a useful source of information about the non-clerical practitioners and their role in society. The Welsh laws suggest that the mediciner was highly ranked, placing him twelfth in order of precedence at the court table; he even lodged with the chief of the household.

The old laws also give some information about their apparatus and medicaments. None of the instruments used by the early Anglo-Saxon and Celtic practitioners have been found. Yet as many of them were probably in common domestic use, they therefore cannot be distinguished. A medicament pan in Welsh law was reckoned to be worth one penny. Medicinal herbs are also known to have been specially cultivated in Wales, as anybody caught stealing them was subject to a special fine payable to the king. Similarly, the Irish invalid was:

to be fed according to the directions of the leech. No person on sick maintenance is entitled in Irish law to any condiment except garden herbs; for it is for this purpose that the gardens have been made, viz. for the care of the sick.

Welsh law also makes provision for protecting the gifts given by a patient to his mediciner from any later claim to wrongful title:

there are three chattels for which no surety is necessary, chattels given by a lord to his man, and a bequest received by a priest from the dead, and chattels received by a physician from a person he attends.

However, the prudent physician would also seek a guarantee from the patient's family that he would not be responsible should the patient "die from the treatment he may give him".

THE LEECH FEE

The Irish and Welsh laws demonstrate some of the stages through which the laws concerning medical practice developed until in the Anglo-Saxon system the physician was paid a separate leech fee.

The Norman Influence On Medical Practice

Edward the Confessor's brother-in-law Harold II was defeated by his cousin William the Conqueror in 1066, with an army of no more than 6,000 men. The Norman Kings, with the aid of some 200 barons, then set about subjugating the kingdom by force. The Domesday Book records that by 1068, with the influx of the Normans, the population of England was one and a half million.

EXISTING MEDICAL PRACTICE IN BRITAIN

On their arrival, the Normans found the best native medicine was practised by the Churchmen, with the support of the Anglo-Saxon leeches. These continued to provide medical care throughout the countryside, but new ideas and practices imported by the conquerors were developed in the royal courts and larger towns.

INFLUENCE OF THE NORMAN CHURCH

There is no evidence of any organised military medical service amongst the Norman Army, and initially the kings relied on the scholarly physicians of the Church, who had crossed from France. Baldwin (d 1097), who was born and educated at Chartres, was such a man and came to England as a direct result of the Norman Conquest. As abbot of Bury St Edmunds, his medical services were in great demand and he was the King's personal physician.

Gilbert Maminot (d 1101), another Norman, was both chaplain and physician to William. He was summoned to attend the King at the Priory of St Gervais near Rouen after the accident in which the King's abdomen was ruptured by the pommel of his saddle when putting his horse to a ditch. After examining his urine, his physicians concluded that death was imminent, but they were so startled by their own accuracy when his end came that they behaved 'like men who had lost their wits'.

John of Villula (d 1122), another Churchman who came to the Conqueror in his last illness, was described by the chronicler William of Malmesbury, as a well-tried physician of more practical experience than scientific knowledge. William Rufus rewarded his services with the bishopric of Wells, and in 1090 he bought the city of Bath from the King, which became the centre of his episcopal see.

Although the majority of the court physicians were Churchmen from France, there was at least one *medicus* in the Conqueror's service, who was not an ecclesiastic. This Nigel, who lived during the latter half of the eleventh century, was a Norman who was rewarded with considerable estates for his medical attendance.

THE ARRIVAL OF OTHER FOREIGN PRACTITIONERS

A number of continental medical practitioners arrived with the

Normans, who brought their own physicians from France. Henry I's wife Matilda was attended at the birth of her first child in 1101 by two Italians when Faritus (d 1117), the abbot of Abbingdon was assisted by Grimaldi (1100–1130), who was already in the royal service. Henry II's *physicus regis* Ralph Bello Monte (or Ralph de Beaumont), drowned in 1171 when part of the royal fleet sank, was also probably Italian.

Most of these physicians of continental origin belonged to the same tradition of medical scholars who had flourished in the monasteries of England and Wales before their destruction by the Danes.

NICHOLAS OF FARNHAM

The chronicler Matthew Paris has provided most of the information available about Nicholas of Farnham, an English practitioner. Nicholas was born in Surrey in the twelfth century, late in the reign of Henry II, and was educated at Oxford and Paris. As was usual in those times, his basic education was in that 'queen of sciences', theology, but he distinguished himself as a teacher and practitioner of medicine at Bologna between 1218 and 1228. He is mentioned as royal physician to King Henry III and Queen Eleanor in 1228. Gifts for his services included benefices, wood, wine, venison, grain and spices. He was more impressive as a physician, however, than he was as a cleric judging by the number of quarrels he had after he was eventually appointed to the bishopric of Durham, where he now lies buried.

Nicholas died in 1257, at Stockton-on-Tees, but before this, believing he was fatally ill, he returned to the south of England to die of 'his uncurable dropsy, discoloured by yellow jaundice, worn away to a skeleton that he might benefit himself by breathing his native air'. He drank some holy water containing a few hairs of St Edmund's beard which made him vomit and 'brought relief from pain and swelling', and he was restored to health. Paris's account of this illness, however, illustrates contemporary medical beliefs which combined the scientific knowledge imported by the foreign physicians, the Anglo-Saxon magic and faith in holy relics.

HOLY RELICS

Faith in the power of the holy relics was shared both by the common people and educated Churchmen in Saxon and Norman times. They believed that the saints in heaven continued to care for earthly men and that the smallest physical remnants of these saints provided a medium through which they could still perform miracles. Many of these relics were of dubious origin. Their claim to authenticity was circumstantial evidence, but this did not dismay those who wished to believe in them.

The bones of Cosmos and Damian, martyred saints of medicine and pharmacy, were said to be amongst the unlikely relics preserved in an iron chest at Canterbury Cathedral; the claim of their presence is made in an inventory of AD 1315, but there is no record of how or when they arrived here from the continent.

HERBALS FROM THE BRITISH MONASTERIES

The British monasteries continued to take an active interest in medicine and science, amongst their other scholarly pursuits. Singer claims that the herbal copies made by monks of the Anglo-Norman period, reached 'the point of lowest illustrational degradation' in the formalised representation of plants which many of the monks had never seen (col. pl. VIII). However, the copyist monk at Baldwin's abbey of Bury St Edmunds broke loose from this slavish tradition to produce naturalistic studies from plants in the monastery garden. Physicians from such monastic houses prepared their own medicines from plants grown in their own herb gardens, and many royal physicians did the same. Those who practised surgery prepared their own dressings, plasters and salves sufficient to keep an adequate stock-in-trade.

Development of the Spicer

OFFICES OF STATE

The great offices of state were beginning to develop in the royal households, although from very humble origins. However, these officers were in a privileged position compared with the harsher realities experienced by the conquered people. Those who became the highest officers of the household considered that their appointment showed a mark of honour. In reality they performed the menial tasks of their office only on feast days when they were richly rewarded. Earl Warenne replaced the ex-communicated Arundel as chief butler at the coronation feast of Queen Eleanor, Henry III's wife, in 1236; he received as his fee the cup with which he served the King. However, those lower down the scale were kept busy all year, and were rewarded in kind and also with robes and money for their work. The Wardrobe, near at hand to the king's person, and associated with the king's comforts, became the office from which such accounts were paid. Originally, next to the king's bedchamber, it acted as a dressing room, a store room and a lavatory, as well as the place where the privy seal for his private accounts was kept.

The steward in charge of the food and wine for the King and royal household, needed to be alert and of proven loyalty in order to guard the king against deliberate poisoning. The master butlers were next in rank to the steward, and beneath them were the master dispensers for bread, the larder and the cellar, and lesser menials under them.

GROWING INTEREST IN SPICES

The purveyor of salt and spices was important in his role to
preserve the food with salt, and disguise ill-preserved food with
spice. The crusades stimulated a special taste for oriental spices,
but all spices, even ordinary pepper, were expensive. The term
'peppercorn rent', which now means a nominal rent, dates from
this time when landlords were glad to accept their rent in the form
of pepper. Fruit and vegetables were of poor quality and meat,
fish and fowl had to be preserved in salt for the winter. The ales
and wines were cloudy and often fermented; sugar was rarely
used as it was scarce and expensive, so honey was used in its place.
King John spent £3 on sugar and spices in 1206, but trade increased
in the thirteenth century when they became more easily available,
although still expensive.

THE OFFICE OF SPICER

The specialised office of spicer to provide spices for food, drugs
and medicine began to appear in the late twelfth century. Initially
he was responsible only for supplying the spices for other people
to use, later he developed into the spicer-apothecary who compounded the syrups, sweetened the electuaries and spiced the
wines.

The first mention of a royal spicer is of a man named William
speciarius regis who served King John in 1207, and remained in
royal service long into Henry III's reign. His main job was to
supply wine, usually at £2 a tun. Elsewhere, there is a record of a
purchase of ale from a merchant called Ralph le Spicer in business
with his wife Amphalissa of London town.

THE ROLE OF THE SPICER OUTSIDE THE ROYAL HOUSEHOLD

As the population became more wealthy there was an increasing
demand for spicers, who began to extend their services beyond
the royal palaces. They imported and sold spices, sugar, wines
and other grocery, and some began to specialise in drugs. The
spicers generated trade with the East and the Italian cities of
Venice, Genoa and Pisa were used as intermediate ports. It is
interesting to note the influence of the spicers in some Italian
words: the modern Italian word for grocer's shop is still *drog-
heria* and the old Italian word for pharmacy was *spezieria* (from
the Latin *species*) indicating the variety of goods sold.

Henry III's merchant Bartholomew the Spicer, lived in a house
in Broad Street in London which was given to his father Joseph
the Spicer, by the King. Bartholomew expanded his business
during Henry's reign, to cater for both the royal household and
the ordinary people.

The bill he presented to the King in 1249 for £93 17s illustrates
the variety of goods he sold; it included silken cloth, rabbits,
almonds and raisins. In 1264 he supplied William, the King's

'sauser', with 20 lb of pepper, half a quarter of cummin and 15 lb of cinnamon and other spices in preparation for the feast of St Edward.

Bartholomew was not a medical man; he sold spices purely for mercenary reasons, and most of his goods were used for culinary, rather than medicinal purposes.

King Henry III had his own spicer, Richard Derkyn who was concerned with the preparation of drugs, and his son John is described as an apothecary. These royal spicer-apothecaries were in charge of the King's spicery and were of a similar rank to the King's serjeants.

ROBERT DE MONTPELLIER

The spicers of Montpellier, a subsidiary centre of the spice trade containing a university destined to play a great part in medical education, also began to practise as apothecaries. One of these spicers, Robert de Montpellier, joined Henry III's service as a *speciarius* in 1243, when the King was visiting Gascony. Robert lived in Milk Street, near the Spiceria of Cheapside, where he became an important tradesman.

There were no fixed boundaries dividing the tasks of the spicer-apothecary and the physician, for the royal physician, Ralph de Neketon, would spice the King's wine in Robert's absence. They worked in close co-operation and between them produced agreeably flavoured medicine. Syrups and sweetened electuaries, which were the consistency of thick paste, were extremely popular; King Edward I's household was supplied with 1,092 lb in 1300, and 165 lb for the Lord Edward himself.

Robert's son Richard continued the family trade as a city spicer, combined with the family appointment of apothecary to the royal household, supplying medicaments and sometimes wine. They sold over £120 of medicaments to Edward I's physician, Nicholas de Tyngewyke (c 1291–1339), during the King's last painful journey north with his army; he was weakened by dysentery and troubled with sore legs. These medicaments included 282 lb of electuaries, ointments, gums, aromatics and plasters.

THE DISTINCTION BETWEEN SPICERS AND APOTHECARIES

Before the thirteenth century, the terms spicer and apothecary were synonymous. Gradually, however, the term spicer came to apply to the general merchant and apothecary to the supplier and compounder of medicines. Spicers, pepperers and grocers continued to congregate near the Spiceria at Cheapside. Those whose interest lay principally in medical treatments collected at Bucklersbury where, in about 1345, they became known as the Fraternity of St Anthony. Even then the distinction was by no means clear cut and the name apothecary was rarely used in the provinces until the fifteenth century.

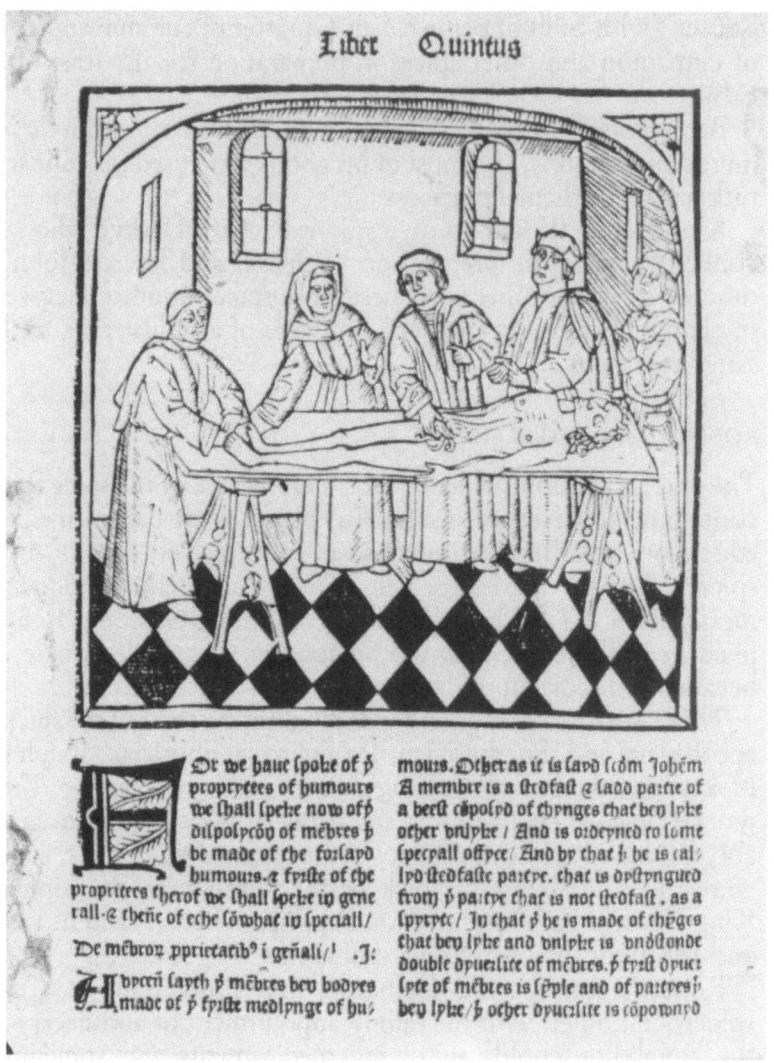

1. A human dissection with a professor demonstrating at the side of the body. It was the first illustration of a dissection to appear in an English book. It appeared in *De Proprietatibus Rerum*, by Bartolomeus Anglicus written in about 1250, and printed by Wynkyn de Worde, Caxton's foreman printer who inherited the press, in 1495.
Reproduced from Singer's Short History of Anatomy, *Dover 1957*.

Other Developments In Medical Practice

SURGICAL TEXTS

Medical works show that far greater advances were made in surgery than medicine at this time, probably because surgical treatment showed more positive results (figure 1). The *Bamberg Surgery* was written at Salerno in the twelfth century; it is mainly a copy of Constantine the African's translation of the Arab Haly Abbas's work, and did not add anything to it. However, Roger of Salerno's *Practica Chirurgia*, later rearranged in a logical sequence by his pupil Guido of Arezzo in 1170, was a great advance on previous works. It eliminated the theorising that weighed down the earlier texts and dealt with surgery in a severely practical manner. Roger describes wound surgery, trepanning, operations for lithotomy, hernia and hydrocele, and he was particularly interested in diagnostic problems.

The *Practica Chirurgia* greatly influenced Gilbertus Anglicus, the only English author of medical importance in the thirteenth century. His *Compendium Medicinae* (c 1240) was of far greater merit than the later and more popular work *Rosa Anglica* (c 1314), by John of Gaddesden. Although Gilbert makes no claim to originality and quotes many sources, he takes an unusually practical and reasonable attitude. He describes diseases in the traditional medieval sequence, beginning with the head and ending with the feet. He includes a particularly good chapter on leprosy, as it was important to possess a knowledge of this disease in the thirteenth century. There is also a passage on women's diseases, illustrated from the text of Trotula, which shows Roger of Salerno's influence. However, Gilbert's description of mental illness illustrates his ability to question traditions by ignoring the popular belief that mental illness was caused by devils.

ORDINARY PRACTITIONERS

These texts influenced the work of medical scholars but the methods of ordinary medical practitioners showed little advance on those of Anglo-Saxon times. The mandrake plant symbolises a continuing belief in magic (col. pl. IX and X). This 'man-shaped' vegetable aphrodisiac had to be torn from the ground by a dog (col. pl. XI) and the dog-handler had to cover his ears for the plant's shriek was fatal, although this precaution never seems to have been recommended for the expendable dog!

5
The Later Plantagenets

The Changing Class Structure

There were 14 Plantagenet kings of England from Henry II (1133–1189) to Richard III (1452–1485). It was a period in which education saw the rise of the universities and in commerce a greater organisation of trade and tradesmen. Before the Battle of Bosworth Field had set the Tudors on the throne in 1485, these developments had left their mark on the medical practitioners.

THE FOUNDATION OF THE UNIVERSITIES

The University of Cambridge was founded in the thirteenth century although it did not receive formal recognition by Pope John XXII until 1318. By the mid fourteenth century the College of Peterhouse had provision for one medical student, Pembroke College had one medical fellow and Gonville College had two. In the fifteenth century, the University established three academic grades in medicine: doctor (MD), baccalaureus (MB), and practicantes in medicine (ML) and surgery or chirurgie (CL). Early records show that the first MD was conferred on James Fries in 1460, and the first MB on Lemster in 1466.

The University of Oxford also issued licences for the practice of medicine and surgery throughout England before 1350. The first Doctorate of Medicine was conferred on Thomas Edmonds in 1449, although previously there had been masters of physic there.

The growth of the medical faculties, and the introduction of degrees and licensing, meant that medical standards were controlled by teachers and examiners. The undergraduates studied medicine only after a general education in the arts faculties, and they developed into a powerful academic elitist class which increasingly dominated the medical profession. They preferred not to treat the poor more often than they could help and this emphasised the gulf between them and the non-academic medical craftsmen (col. pl. XII).

In 1421, during the reign of Henry V, the older universities petitioned Parliament to restrict the practice of physic to those who had graduated. Parliament also included the small but select group of surgeons who had 'trained for surgery with the masters of that art' in its attempt to separate the 'cunning from the uncunning'. The avowed purpose was to make it known that:

many uncunning and unapproved in the foresaid Science practises, and especially in Physic, so that in this Realm is every man, be he never so lewd, taking upon him practise, be suffered to use it, to great harm and slaughter of many men: Where if no man practised therein but all only cunning men and approved sufficiently learned in art, philosophy and physic, as it is kept in other lands and realms, there should many men that dies, for default of help, life, and no man perishes by uncunning.

This was the first attempt to provide a medical register so that laymen could distinguish those who were considered safe practitioners by the profession and the government. However, it was not made into a statute and the Privy Council had no power to enforce it. It did not prevent the country folk from consulting those neighbours who were willing to help them with advice and treatment for their ailments. It was not until the Tudors came to the throne that the profession became regulated by statute.

THE RISE OF THE MERCHANT CLASS

The fourteenth century was marked by the struggle of people to improve their status. This was particularly evident in the merchant class. They aspired to become part of the aristocracy, a transition made easier by the acquisition of money. Money blurred distinctions of rank and in the wool trade it was not unusual for shopkeepers and warehouse owners of one generation to become lords of the manor in the next. Similarly, it was possible to capitalise on the king's need to borrow money to finance wars. Although this ruined many speculators, those who were sufficiently astute could succeed in pleasing the king, while also founding their own fortunes and bettering their positions.

This struggle for wealth and social standing consequently produced richer medical practitioners. The surgeon and apothecary, providing medical care for the merchant class, shared in its new found prosperity, while also fighting to better their place in the social scale.

MEDICAL CARE FOR THE COMMON PEOPLE

The majority of the population was cared for by a group of practitioners who were in the tradition of the Anglo-Saxon leeches. These people were mainly local villagers who had some knowledge of herbal lore and nursing skill.

Despite the differences between the medical practitioners caring for the various classes of society, they were generally all alike in their lack of specialisation. The main division between them was marked by a leaning towards either surgery, as in the surgeon-apothecaries, or medicine, which was favoured by the new graduates.

CLERICAL PRACTITIONERS

In principle the papal authorities became strongly opposed to the practice of medicine by the *religiosi*. In 1130 the fifth canon of the Council of Clermont declared that monks and canons regular, having donned the habit and taken vows, were no longer to study medicine or law for financial gain, or act as lawyers or physicians. The repetition of these injunctions suggests that members of the clergy were often tempted to practise medicine for money. This necessitated monks leaving their monastery, against the rule binding them to stay within its confines. The Fourth Lateran Council in 1215, under Pope Innocent III, specifically forbade any surgery which involved using the knife or cautery. These operations were only a small part of the surgeon's work which also included the treatment of fractures, dislocations, eye disease and skin disease. The injunction was repeated by Boniface VIII in 1298.

The Church provided medical care for sick monks, and this service was later extended to lay brothers and pilgrims. Some monasteries also developed specialised services which included facilities for lepers, the mentally ill and the confinement of pregnant women.

The Development of the Gilds

THE NEED FOR GILDS

With the growth of trade in the thirteenth and fourteenth centuries, the merchants began to unite into companies which furthered their business and protected their interests. This trend was encouraged by the King and nobility who felt that an organised citizenry could be governed more effectively by them. It was the crisis in the agricultural economy in the 1360s, associated with the Black Death, which persuaded the King of the need for further control. In 1349, the Ordinance of Labourers had sought to control the wages and movement of labour, but without much success. In 1363, Edward III decreed that all tradesmen and craftsmen, *gentz de meistere*, must belong to a gild, although it did not have to be a gild of their own trade or craft.

THE RELIGIOUS, MERCHANT AND CRAFT GILDS

By the fourteenth century there were three distinct varieties of gilds: the religious, the merchant and the craft gilds. The religious gilds were similar to the modern friendly societies. The merchant gilds, which were of much older origin than the religious gilds, created and protected a monopoly in a particular trade. Some of the merchant gilds had a broad membership from which specialist groups later split off to form their own craft gilds. These craft gilds required that all their members should reach a particular standard and they also laid down rules which governed apprenticeships to their trades. It was through these gilds that the apothecary eventually became organised as a medical practitioner, and the barber-surgeon's skill was acknowledged.

The number of non-academic practitioners, which included apothecaries, spicer-apothecaries, surgeon-apothecaries, barber-surgeons and surgeons, had been growing from the beginning of the fourteenth century. In London, both the Gild of Surgeons and the Company of Barbers looked after the welfare of the surgeons and their apprentices. The Company of Barbers, unlike the Gild of Surgeons, had a very broad membership of physicians, surgeons, apothecaries, silk weavers, chandlers and rope-makers.

THE GROCERS' COMPANY

In 1345, pepperers, grocers and apothecaries came together as the Gild of St Anthony. The Grocers' Company from which the Society of Apothecaries was to spring, was given its Charter in 1429. This Company was always willing to co-operate with the Plantagenets over money and most of its revenue came from the charge of the King's Beam, upon which the heavy merchandise imported into the City of London was weighed. This was granted to the Company in 1383 by Richard II, and its name derives from this method of charging: *grossarii* means those who sell by weight.

The Grocers' Company included pepperers, spicers and apothecaries, and in 1456 Henry VI gave them the right to garble drugs and spices, so that these could be classified and certified free from adulteration. With the gradual separation of medicine from grocery, the right to 'enter, view and search' passed to the physicians and later to the apothecaries.

THE COMPETITION BETWEEN THE GILDS

The power of a gild was in direct proportion to the number of its members, and therefore there was intense competition between them to increase their membership. While the Grocers' Company gained control over the apothecaries during the Plantagenet period, the battle for the surgeons was being fought out in London between the Company of Surgeons and the Company of Barber-Surgeons. However, the Barbers' Company had the numerical advantage and when the royal charter was granted in 1462, it was sufficiently powerful to ensure the support of the Surgeons.

This power struggle was not reflected in the provinces where there were insufficient surgeons and apothecaries in any one town

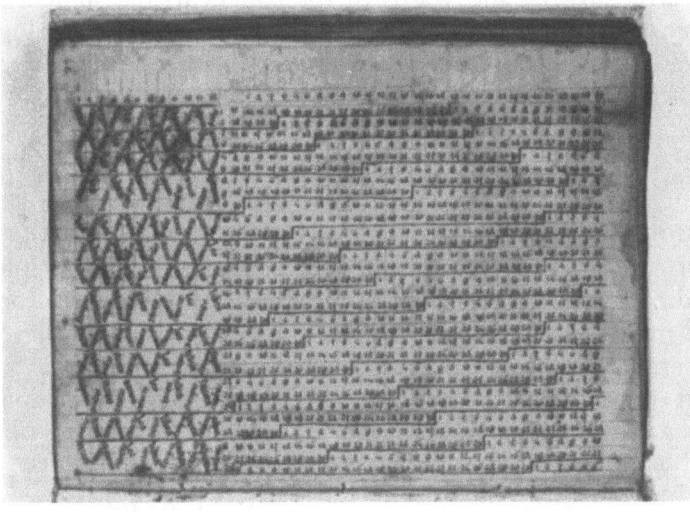

1. A table used in astrological medicine. From the fifteenth century Mostyn MS 88.
By courtesy of the National Library of Wales.

to make the dispute of much importance. The practitioners were content to remain members of one of the merchant gilds such as a Grocers' Gild or Mercers' Gild, or a Barber-Surgeons' Company.

THE COMPETITION BETWEEN THE ACADEMIC AND NON-ACADEMIC PRACTITIONERS

The academic physicians remained aloof from the apothecaries, their non-academic counterparts, and similarly the surgeons strongly resented the power of the barbers. The academic practitioners considered that they were superior both by education and class, and this power struggle delayed the rational cohesion of the medical profession.

Other Medical Developments

MEDICAL LITERATURE

John of Arderne (1307–1392) was a surgeon who was trained by his service in the army, and in 1370 became a member of the Gild of Barber-Surgeons. His writings on surgery were collected as his *Practica,* in which he advocates cleanliness and condemns pus-forming salves. He commanded large fees, particularly for his operation which laid open the anal fistula. For this operation, he demanded £40 down, a suit of clothes and £5 annually for the patient's lifetime.

Caxton introduced printing into England in 1474 which increased the availability of medical literature. John of Gaddesden's work *Rosa Anglica* of 1314 was first printed in 1492 in Pavia and went through many editions to become one of the most widely used medical treatises of the later Middle Ages. It was compiled from many earlier writings and gives an overall view of continental medicine in the previous two centuries. He stresses the importance of taking a good medical case history. He takes a practical attitude towards surgery and warns of the danger to the sphincter ani when treating the fistula, 'lest after the cure there arise involuntary release of the faeces'. He also preferred the use of the truss to the knife in treating herniae, as did many later surgeons.

ASTROLOGY

Astrology played an important part in the medical practice of the fourteenth, fifteenth and sixteenth centuries. The principles of medical astrology were linked with the hypothesis of microcosm and macrocosm. The planets, or inner circles, were believed to govern man's internal organs, while the zodiac, or external belt of stars, related to his surface anatomy. This astrological relationship was a development of Aristotle's concept of microcosm or man and his internal behaviour, and macrocosm or the universe and the movements of the external heavens (see page 47).

Microcosm and macrocosm were made up of the four primary elements: earth, fire, air and water. Each of these elements contained a pair of the four qualities: hot, cold, wet and dry, which were also combined in the associated humours: blood, black bile, yellow bile and phlegm. One humour predominated in each of the four temperaments: sanguine, melancholic, choleric and phlegmatic.

Many diagrams were made showing the zodiacal signs in relation to the human body (col. pl. XIII). Later, diagrams of venous man aided the practice of blood letting by including instructions on where to bleed for different complaints (col. pl. XIV). The choice of site was important as the blood system was believed to be ebbing and flowing, which was the galenical theory, rather than circulatory.

It was necessary to use astrological tables in conjunction with the diagrams, and by the end of the fourteenth century, ingenious ready-reckoners had been devised for 'instant' bedside diagnosis (figures 1 and 2). Urine-gazing was an established means of diagnosing illness, and *vade mecums* often contained a roundel of urine flasks showing the significance of the different colours. Many of these tables, calendars and diagrams were produced by the stationers of the Middle Ages as basic outline plans for completion by individual practitioners.

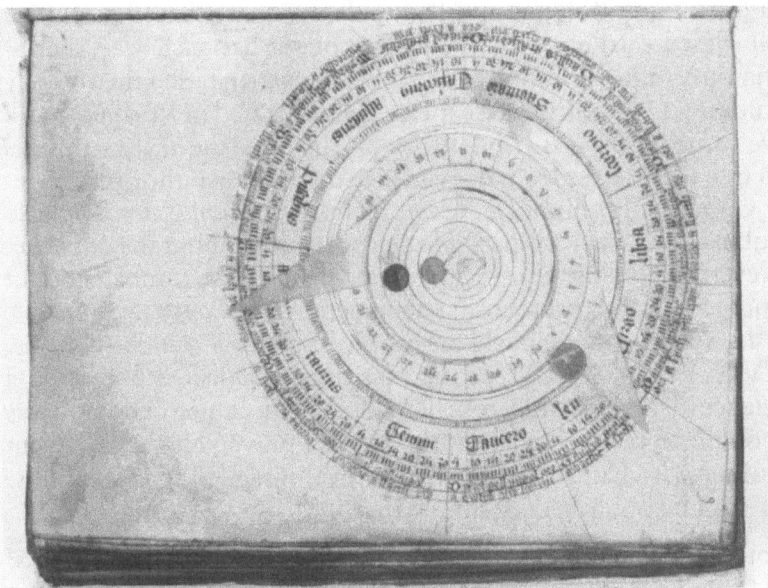

2. A moveable calculator used in astrological medicine. From the fifteenth century Mostyn MS 88. *By courtesy of the National Library of Wales.*

6
The Tudors

The New Interest in Education

In 1485, with the emblem of the Red Dragon flying at Bosworth Field, Henry Tudor took the throne of England. The Welsh dynasty was one of promise for the country, whose kings and queens were to give encouragement for their subjects to take part in a national adventure. It was a time of self-made men, a time when education could better a man's position:

As for gentlemen, they be made good cheape in England. For whosoever studieth the lawes of the realme, who studieth in the universities, who professeth liberall sciences, and to be shorte, who can live idly and without manuall labour, and will beare the port, charge and countenaunce of a gentleman, he . . . shall be taken for a gentleman.

A new type of aristocracy began to develop. The more ambitious were attracted to the court of London where they competed for position and its high rewards.

THE NEW LEARNING

The Italian Renaissance encouraged the exchange of scholars among different universities. Many British students took the opportunity to complete their education on the continent and to distinguish themselves by contacts with the international centres of learning in Bologna and Padua. It was there that they studied the New Learning, with its emphasis on the basic sciences, such as anatomy, and the importance of observing man rather than merely studying textbooks. These ideas, demonstrated in Vesalius' work *De Fabrica Corporis Humani* in 1543, inspired the new anatomists to free themselves from dependence on written authority.

Copernicus's book *De Revolutionibus Orbium Celestium*, also published in 1543, disproved ancient theories about the universe. Nevertheless, the use of astrology in medicine, and tenets of microcosm and macrocosm still lingered on.

In 1542 Leonard Fuchs in his *De Historia Stirpium* (col. pls. XV, XVI and XVII), for the first time established botany as a science distinguishable from herb lore. The teaching of botany was thought to be inadequate at the English universities and William Turner who had studied at Cambridge, intended to correct this. In 1548 he published a guide so that:

Potecaries shoulde be excuselesse when as the ryghte herbes are required of them, I have showed in what places of Englande, Germany and Italy the herbes growe and maye be had for laboure and money.

In 1551, he started his *New Herball* which contained some original material, although many illustrations were taken from Fuchs, and it is by this work that he became known as the father of English botany.

The New Medicine emphasised the importance of the basic sciences. There were no comparable advances in diagnosis and

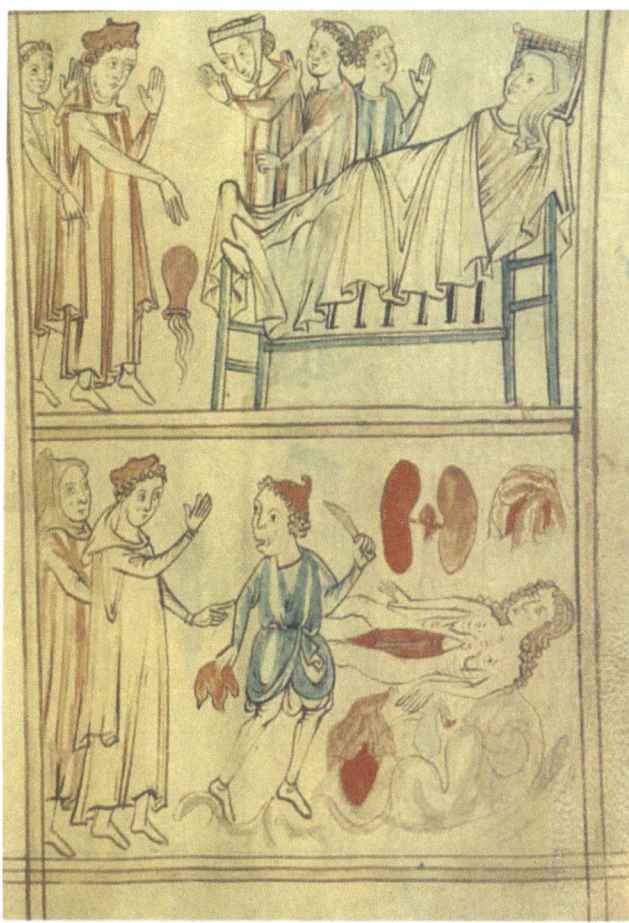

XII
(Above) A sick lady with her physician. The dropped urine flask indicates that the condition is hopeless. (Below) The patient has died and a post-mortem is in progress. Thirteenth century. From the Ashmole MS 399 folio 34.
By courtesy of the Bodleian Library.

XIII
The Zodiac Man. The signs of the zodiac are shown in relation to the body. The Welsh instructions indicate times for avoiding venesection at particular sites. From the fifteenth century Mostyn MS 88.
By courtesy of the National Library of Wales.

XIV
The Welsh Bleeding Man. The instructions in the circles indicate the diseases best treated by bleeding at those sites. The medical artist seems to have had a sense of humour, because the translation for the armpits suggests that if bled here the patient will die from laughing. From the fifteenth century Mostyn MS 88.
By courtesy of the National Library of Wales.

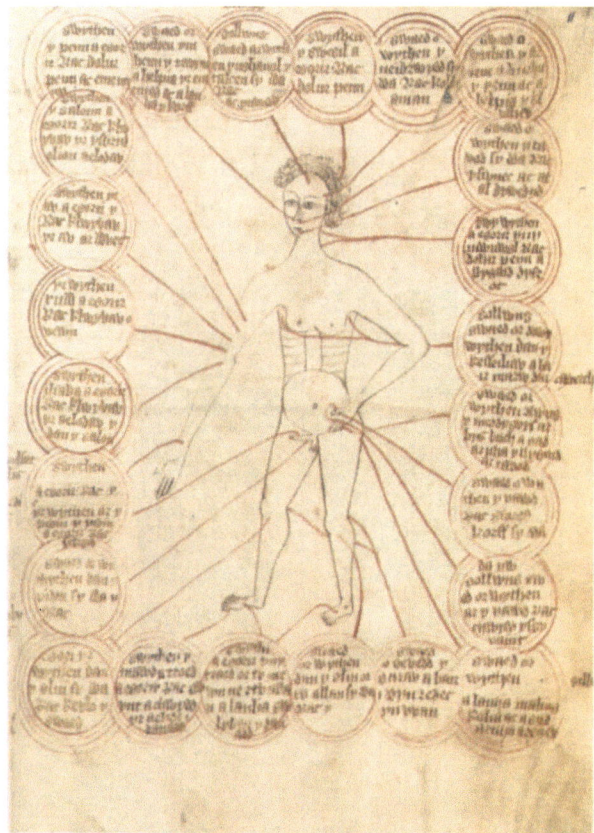

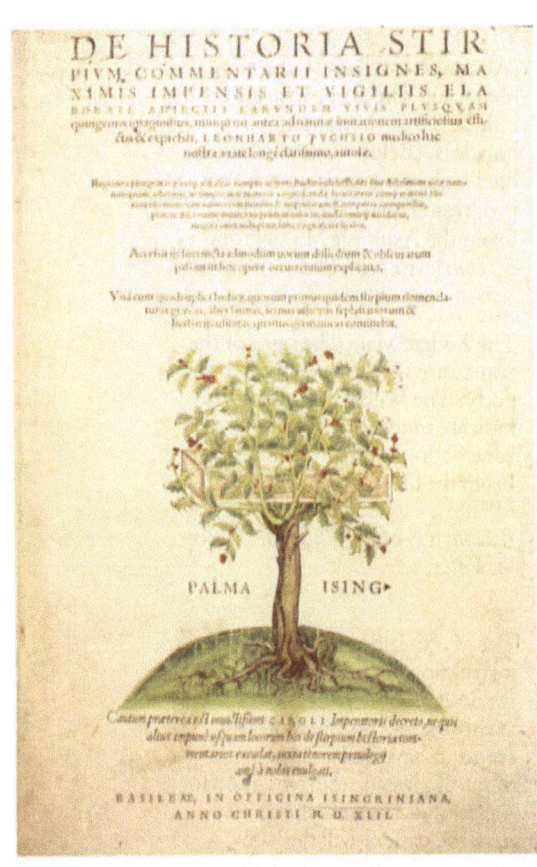

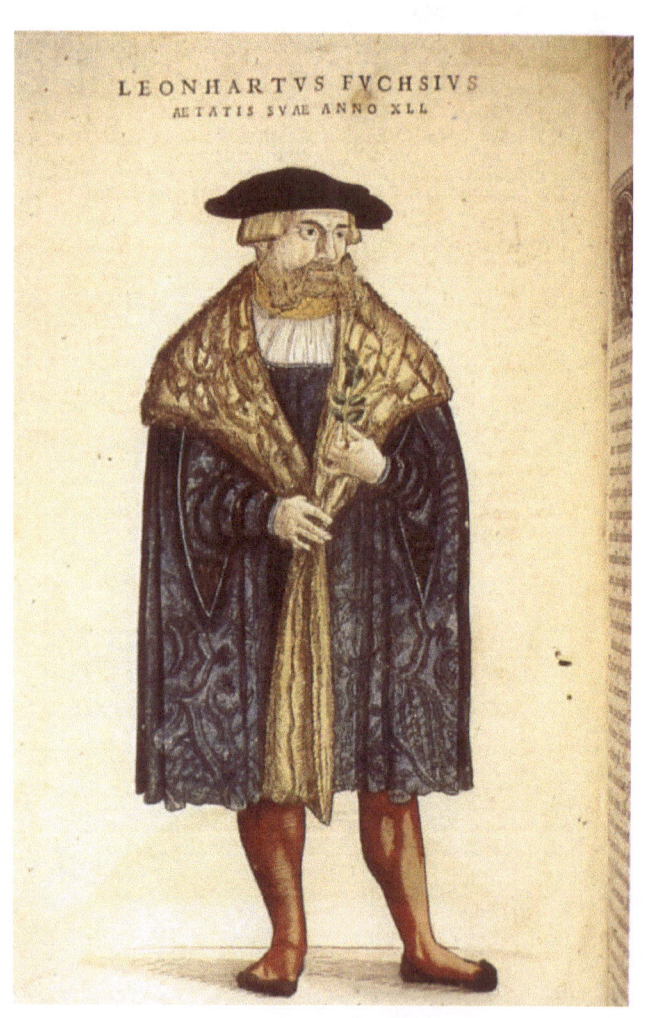

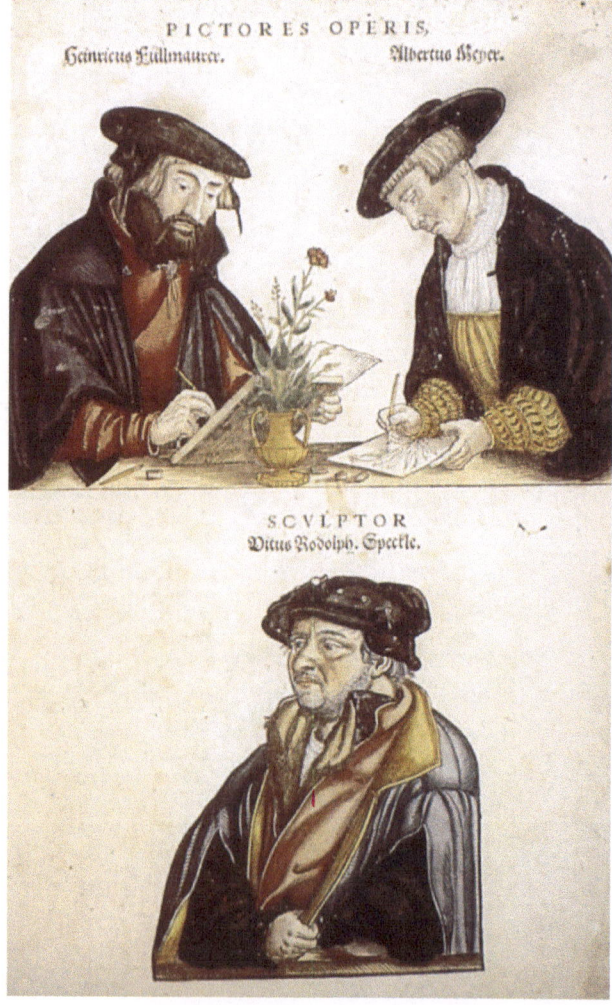

XV
The title page of *De Historia Stirpium* by Leonard Fuchs.
By courtesy of the Wellcome Trustees.

XVI
Leonard Fuchs, *De Historia Stirpium*.
By courtesy of the Wellcome Trustees.

XVII
Portraits in *De Historia Stirpium* of Heinrich Füllmaurer and Albrecht Meyer, who drew the plants for Fuchs' book, and Rodolph Speckle the engraver. These are the earliest portraits of scientific illustrators.
By courtesy of the Wellcome Trustees.

treatment, unfortunately, and the medical profession had to rely on the old practices, even though based on theories which had been disproved.

MEDICAL SYLLABUS AT THE UNIVERSITIES

The Statuta Antiqua had hitherto governed the medical syllabus at Cambridge and Oxford. A preliminary training in the arts, preceding the study of medicine, was regarded as necessary to produce an educated man. The medical training itself was based on Galen (see page 51), and both Thomas Linacre (1466–1524) and John Caius (1510–1573) devoted their lives to translating and editing his works. The regius professor, first appointed at Cambridge in 1540, and Oxford in 1546, had the duty of reading Hippocrates and Galen four days a week. He also performed one dissection a year, which was but a demonstration of the text of Galen, and this was only carried out at the students' request.

Initially, the New Learning was accessible only to those people who could travel to foreign universities, but with the introduction of printing, the works of Vesalius (figures 1, 2 and 3), Copernicus and Fuchs became more widely available in Britain. The students at the universities complained that they had little time to study the New Learning, as their curriculum was so overcrowded with non-medical subjects. The universities became increasingly aware of the need to set a new medical syllabus, and limit the subjects studied, if they were to produce scholars of the New Science. As a result, the Elizabethan Statutes for the University were introduced in 1570; they established medicine as an independent subject not requiring a preliminary training in the arts. Candidates had to

1. Plates from Vesalius' muscle man arranged as a frieze to show the Paduan hills in the background. The plates are printed as mirror images, as originally drawn for the 1543 and 1555 editions. From the *Fifth Centenary Jubilee Celebrations of Basle University* by F. Hoffmann, La Roche & Co. Published 1960.
By courtesy of the Wellcome Trustees.

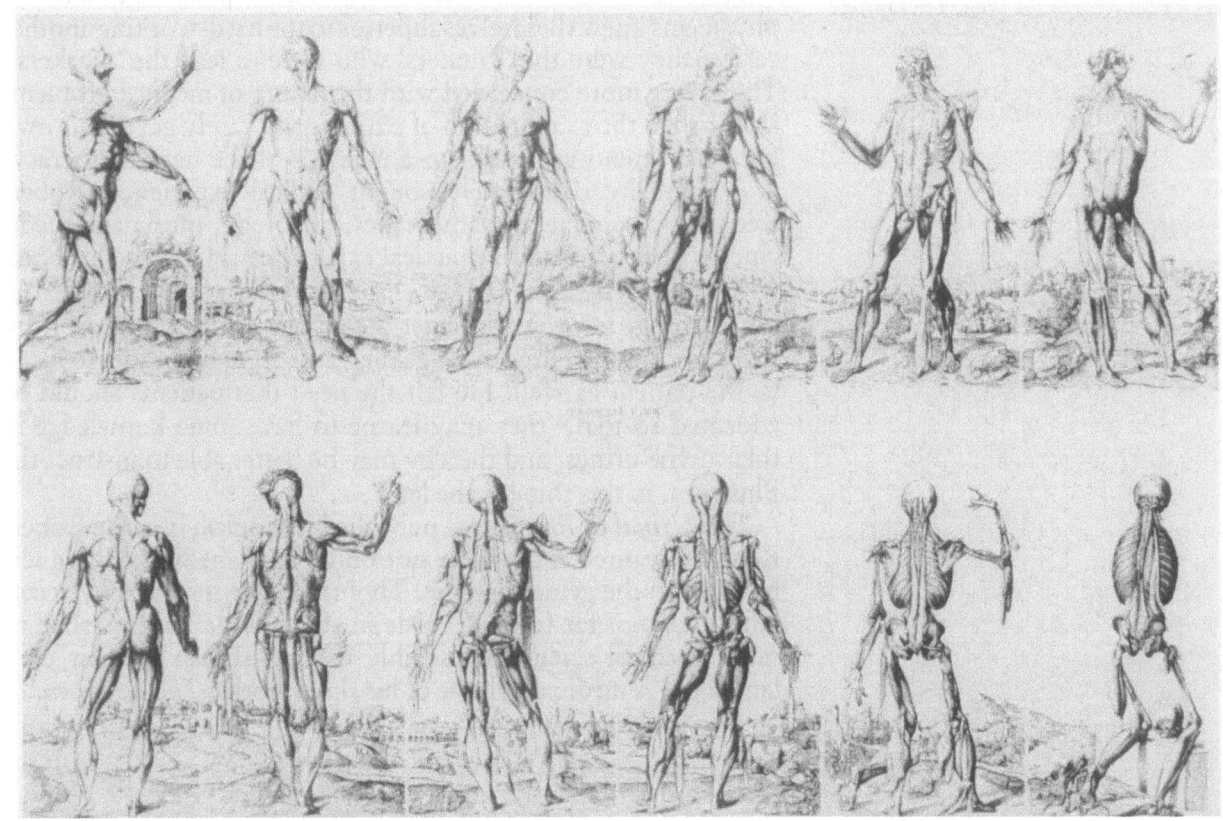

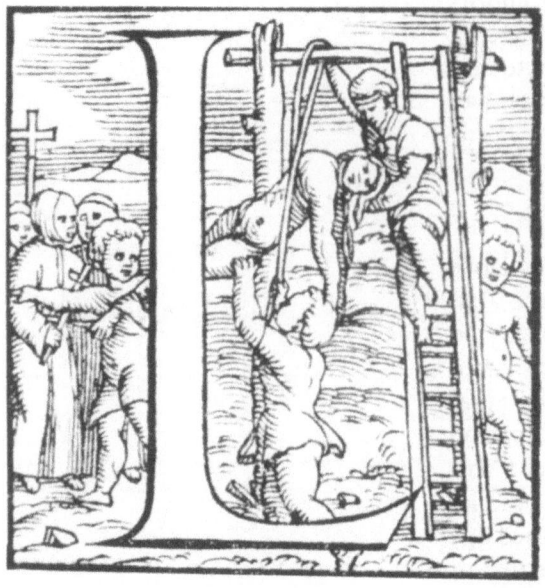

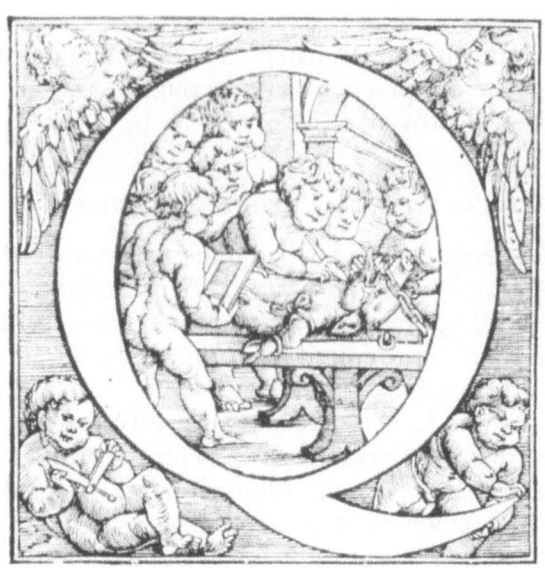

2. Vesalius' initial letter 'L'. The illustration shows the body of a hanged felon being removed from the gallows for dissection. The body appears to be that of a woman. From Andreas Vesalius' *De Humani Corporis Fabrica*, Basle 1555. *By courtesy of the Wellcome Trustees.*

3. Vesalius' initial letter 'Q'. The illustration shows cherubs dissecting a living pig fastened to a dissection board. From Andreas Vesalius' *De Humani Corporis Fabrica*, Basle 1555. *By courtesy of the Wellcome Trustees.*

have seen two dissections and taken part in three disputations in the schools. The pattern of medical teaching was then set for the next 300 years.

Hierarchy of the Medical Profession

UNIVERSITY EDUCATED PHYSICIANS

A belief in the natural order of things, the chain of being, was firmly held by the people of the Middle Ages and it was natural for them to accept any hierarchy whether it was in the social structure, government or medical profession.

The universities flourished under Tudor patronage, and the physicians knew themselves superior to the hard-working apothecaries; they were the 'thinkers' who were to lead the 'workers'. They were more concerned with the nature of medical problems rather than the examination of patients and rarely gave their own personal attention, except to a member of the new aristocracy.

A minority deliberately sought clinical experience. Robert Recorde, a scholar of mathematics, astrology, music and medicine, was also a man of practical experience. He wrote his book *Urinal of Physic*, 1547 (figure 4), so that others might profit from his learning. He warns against the dangers of detachment from the patient, inherent in urine gazing, and urges the reader to listen to the patient as well! He felt the need that patients should be educated so that, 'they may learne to have some knowledge in their owne urines, and thereby may be better able to instruct the Phisition, in this thing at the least . . .'

The *Urinal of Physic* was published in English because Robert Recorde wanted it available not only to his medical colleagues, but also to the general public. Thomas Phaer another physician, who lived not far from Recorde in south Wales, also wished to make medical science intelligible to Englishmen in their own language. A medical volume of his three works, *The Regiment of*

40

Life, A Treatise of the Pestilence and *The Booke of Children*
(figure 5) was published in 1545.

Generally, the physicians used the local apothecary as an intermediary, first to give a history of the case and then to carry out the prescribed treatment. Such physicians and apothecaries usually worked amicably together: this is illustrated by a letter from William Goldwyn a physician, to John Byrell, an apothecary, concerning the treatment of Lady Stonor:

Syr, I recommende me unto yow, praying yow as hertely as I may that
ye have over syghte in the servyng of thys byll, as my truste ys in yow:
for thys ys for a specyall Mastres of myn. And with the grace of God hit
schall not be longe or I see yow. And then I purpose for to tary with yow.

The apothecaries soon learnt that they could diagnose and treat
without the physician's interference. The physicians then saw
them as a threat to their livelihood and therefore strongly resisted
such attempts to usurp their role.

THE APOTHECARIES

The apothecaries, apothecary-surgeons, surgeons and barber-surgeons comprised the main body of medical and surgical practitioners in London. They were becoming increasingly important in the social scale, and the apothecaries in particular had been encouraged in their social aspirations by royal patronage. Thomas Alsop became chief apothecary to Henry VIII and was given the title of Gentleman Apothecary. The King also took an interest in practical pharmacy and Sloan MS 1047 contains many formulae which are attributed to him.

Apothecaries were in constant demand by the wealthy who wanted dragees, perfumes, spices and confectionery. Matthews the pharmaceutical historian, describes the frequency with which 'dredge cumfytts' or sugar-coated sweets appeared in the apothecaries' bills.

The apothecaries also made up prescriptions for the physicians and supplied them with drugs; they made electuaries with confection of barberry, plasters of *unguentum rosarum et infrigidans gallen* (or Galen's cold cream), and supplied guiacum, Venice treacle and mithridatium (figure 6). In June 1589, the College of Physicians decided to compile a pharmacopoeia for the use of apothecaries, which included salts, chemicals and metals in its headings. The *Pharmacopoeia Londinensis* of 1618, was derived from this. Herb remedies, known as simples or galenicals, were becoming increasingly popular and there were numerous printed herbals. Dr Bullein felt that all good apothecaries should have their own gardens with plenty of 'herbs, seeds and roots', and physic gardens for the exclusive production of medicinal herbs were becoming more common. John Gerard, who published a herbal in 1597, grew the plants he describes in a garden at Holborn.

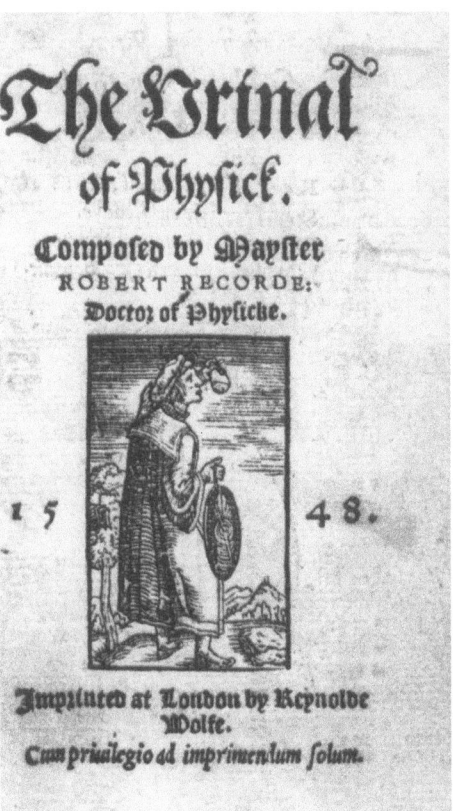

4. The title page of Robert Recorde's
Urinal of Physic, 1548 edition.
*By courtesy of the National Library of
Wales.*

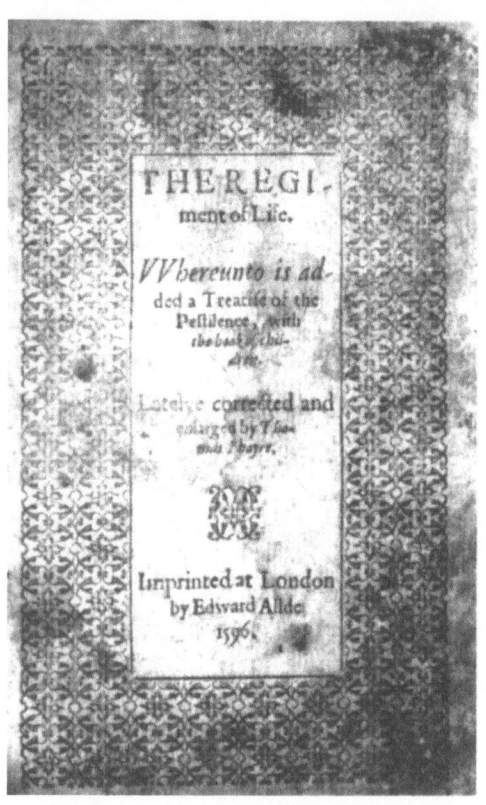

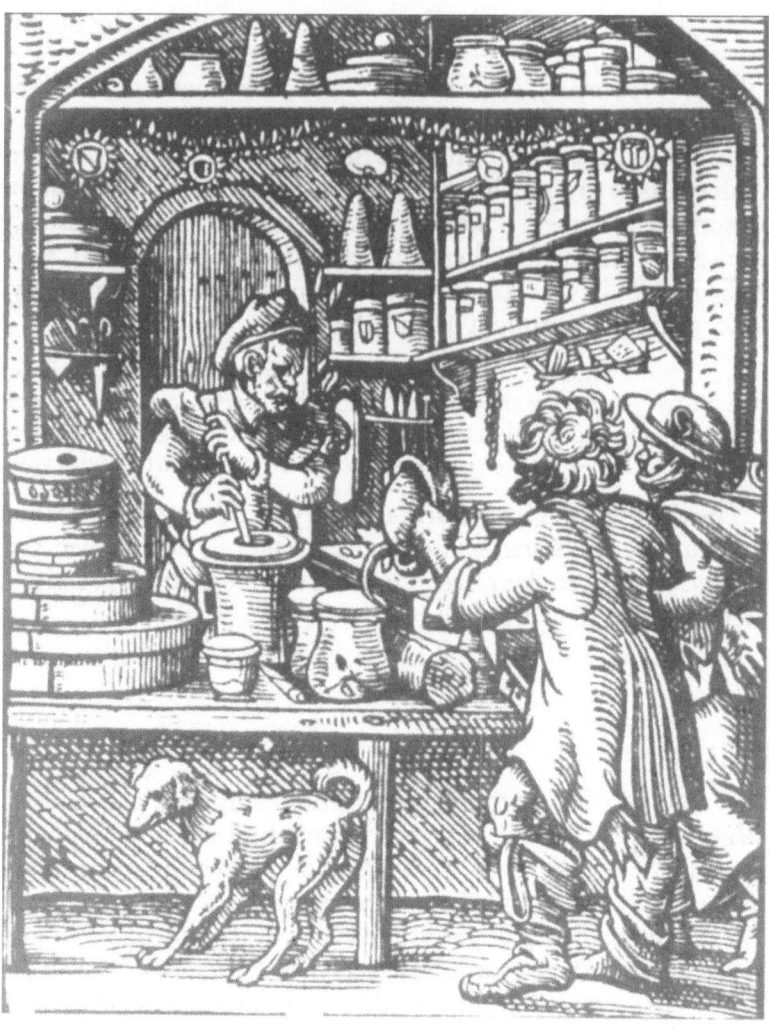

5. The title page of *The Regiment of Life – The Book of Children*, Edwarde Allde edition 1596, by Thomas Phaer. *By courtesy of the National Library of Wales.*

6. An apothecary's shop in 1568. *Reproduced from* Doctors and Disease in Tudor Times *by W. S. C. Copeman, published by Dawsons.*

UNQUALIFIED PRACTITIONERS

Many apothecaries and surgeons were fully occupied looking after the merchant class and did not wish to lower their social standing and income by providing medical care for the poor. This lower class had therefore to be looked after by unqualified practitioners, and local herbalists, and sometimes by itinerant quacks and other charlatans (figure 7).

The inhabitants of the great country houses often made and dispensed their own home remedies, aided by books written for the layman, such as Sir Thomas Elyot's *Castle of Health* (c 1536), Andrew Boord's *Breviary of Helthe* (1547) and *Compendyous Regimente or Dyetary of Health* (1542).

Attempts to Control Medical Practice

THE ACT OF 1512

The Plantagenets had attempted to control the practice of medicine in 1421 but they never had the force of law (see page 32). Henry VIII was anxious to prevent untrained, unorganised and sometimes unscrupulous practitioners abusing the welfare of his subjects. In 1512 he introduced an Act with which he hoped to

42

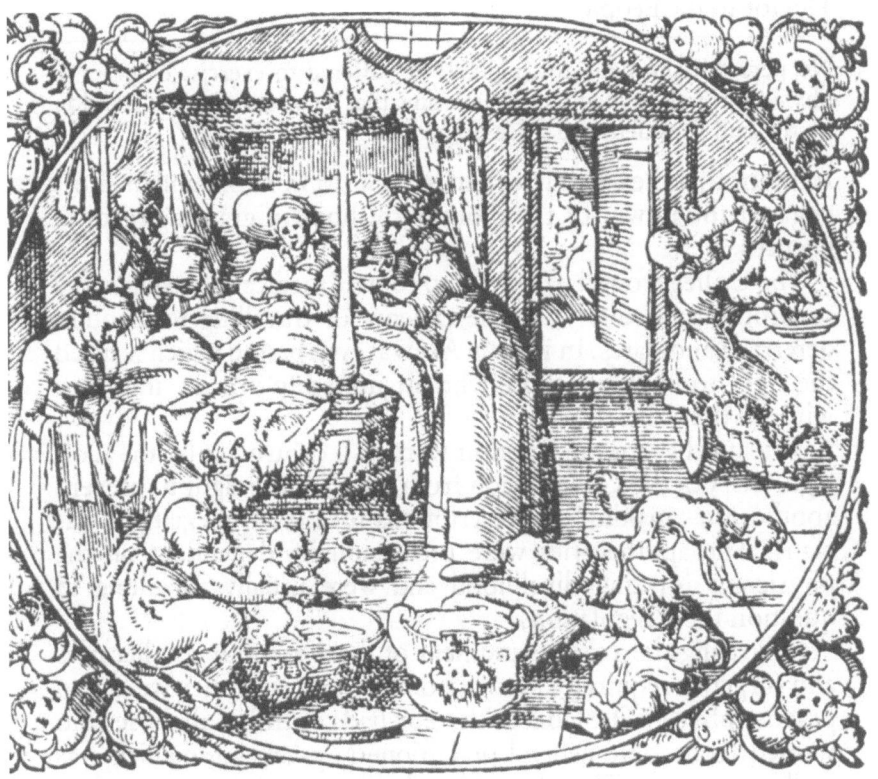

control medical practice through regional administration, without imperilling the supply of practitioners. The Church had been associated with caring for the sick and already had a diocesan organisation, so the Act recommended that licences to practise should be granted by the diocesan bishops. The licences were to enable the public to recognise a competent practitioner and the bishops were to be guided by an examining panel of either practising physicians or surgeons.

Licences were granted separately for medicine and surgery. In 1514, William Ashewell, barber surgeon was licensed to practise surgery by Richard FitzJames, Bishop of London, 'with thassistance of John Smyth doctour of physicke,' and, 'iiii experte persons in the faculte of Surgery after the tenor of the saide art'.

THE COLLEGE OF PHYSICIANS

Thomas Linacre founded the College of Physicians in London in 1518. The foundation charter of the College, granted by Henry VIII, gave it the right to limit the practice of medicine, within seven miles of London, to those licensed by the College. The bishops had experienced difficulty in finding enough physicians outside London to fill their examining boards so the College charter was extended in 1523 to enable the College to grant licences to practise medicine throughout the whole of England, exempting only those who were graduates of Oxford or Cambridge.

This extension of the Act in 1523, permitted the College to reject candidates without the qualifications deemed necessary by the president:

7. A sixteenth century lying-in scene from a woodcut on the title page of the seventeenth century Dutch editions of *De Conceptu et Generatione Hominis* by Jacob Reuff.
Reproduced by permission of Oxford University Press from A Short History of Medicine *by Singer and Ashworth.*

No person from henceforth [shall] be suffered to exercise or practise physic through England until such time that he be examined at London by the said President and three of the Elects' of the College.

It meant that the candidates had to come to London, and in effect negated the power of the diocesan bishops in granting medical licences.

The College found it difficult to control medical licensing in the provinces particularly, as the expense of travelling to London deterred candidates. In 1553 an Act was even passed which secured the right to imprison those who attempted to practise medicine without the College licence.

The apothecaries in London were also controlled by the College. In 1524 the College won from the City the right to prevent apothecaries making up prescriptions for non-Collegiate physicians. The apothecaries were professionally dependent on the physicians for their livelihood and were usually unwilling to question these regulations.

Following the 1523 amendment of the Act, both apothecaries and surgeons required a licence from the College if they wished to practise physic. The College thereby had control of all those who wished to become general practitioners, practising medicine as well as surgery. The physicians themselves were permitted to practise surgery without further licence.

The College of Physicians, through these different Acts, established its control over medicine. No more than a dozen physicians were attempting to enforce an exclusive right to treat a population of 60,000 people in London alone.

SURGEONS

The College was content to allow the Church to continue its power over the surgeons, to which the chartered surgeons strongly objected. They have been described as illiterate, but many read surgical works and collected books and manuscripts. William Witwang (c 1478–1501), citizen and surgeon of London, made bequests in his will of his 'grete boke of phisik and surgery', and 'the residue of all my books of Englisshe and Laten'.

Surgeons such as Thomas Gale (1507–1587), William Clowes (1540–1604) and John Woodall (1569–1643) also recorded their methods of practice and their results. Most of their works are devoted to gunshot wounds, burns and amputations, with some interest in the new disease of syphilis. Woodall, in the *Surgeon's Mate* (1639) advocates the use of limes and lemons in the prophylaxis of scurvy. He also gives a detailed account of circular amputation, 'Six (men) and not fewer are the least for taking off a member proceeding by a wound by gunshot'.

English translations of works by continental surgeons were also available. Giovanni da Vigo's *Surgery* (1543) introduced the theory that gunpowder was poisonous and treated gunshot wounds with boiling oil. Ambroise Paré (1510–1590), however, had the common sense to see that this simply made matters worse, and helped the barbarous practice to die out. These books by foreign surgeons also contained many remedies for ulcers and skin diseases, and advice on purging, cupping and blistering. Tents made of soft vegetable matter or linen were used to keep wounds open for drainage, and a seton of thread or bristle would be drawn through a sinus to keep open its orifice.

The barber-surgeons objected to the power of the bishops to give licences which diminished their hard-won rights granted by their royal charter in 1462 (col. pl. XVIII). Despite their appeals, the bishops retained this privilege.

Before granting licences, the bishops were required to see that candidates should be examined by experienced gild surgeons. Unfortunately, the bishops' officers did not always check the examiners' findings. These licences were not always backed up by an examiner's certificate of competence, and lowered the standard of practice.

In 1540 the surgeons were eventually allowed to form the United Company of Barber-Surgeons, but this company only had the power to control surgery within one mile of the City.

THE GROWING DEMAND FOR GENERAL PRACTITIONERS

Despite the efforts of the College of Physicians to separate medicine and surgery, a new class of practitioners developed, practising both branches of medicine. It was obviously in the patient's interest to find a practitioner who was competent in both disciplines. He was likely to be an apothecary or surgeon, either of whom had more practical experience than the physician.

The surgeons, who made their own salves and plasters, saw no reason why they should not also give internal remedies for patients under their care. They personally treated a wide range of ailments including abscesses, injuries, skin diseases (including syphilis – the New Disease – with mercury), the plague, sweating sickness and tumours. Leprosy had virtually disappeared by this time. Balthazar de Gracys, a London surgeon of the early years of the sixteenth century, claimed to have cured Alexander Marten of the great pox 'savying that he leffte a litell issue to be runnyng in oon of his lygges for the preservacion of his lyff'. Many of these surgeons had served in the army or navy and therefore had experience of treating the illnesses with which soldiers and sailors were afflicted.

Unlike the apothecaries, the surgeons were not so subordinated to the physicians and they were far bolder in defying the College. The surgeons often had much wider experience of medical practice and usually it was the surgeon who took the role of the Tudor general practitioner. In 1575, John Banester, an anatomist surgeon (col. pl. XIX), published *A Needefull, New and Necessarie Treatise of Chyrurgerie* advocating the unity of physic and surgery. He followed this with *A Compendious Chyrurgerie* in 1585.

THE ADVERSE RESULTS OF THE LICENSING ACTS

The legislation governing the issue of licences to medical practitioners had several serious drawbacks. It could have deprived many people of any form of medical care and subjected many who did practise to harassment. The College of Physicians used the Acts to strengthen its own position. Surgeons, apothecaries and non-Collegiate physicians had no legal status as general practitioners unless both their certificates were in order. If not, they were liable to prosecution by either the physicians or surgeons, with a fine of £10 a month. Half of this fine was paid to the informers, who were naturally not hard to find!

In 1542, therefore, an Act was passed which was designed to protect the herbalist, non-qualified practitioners and 'divers honest persons . . . whom God hath endued with the knowledge of the nature, kind and operation of certain herbs, roots, and waters, and the using and ministering of them . . .' It permitted them to 'minister in and to any outward sore' and to 'give drinks for the stone'. It was a well-meaning compromise to try to keep the balance and became unfairly known as the 'Quacks' Charter'.

By the sixteenth century, the philosophical basis had been developed to a point where further progress in diagnosis and treatment was simply not possible just by the continuing and relentless application of unrelieved thoughtful theory alone. It was not that the medical philosophers were running out of ideas. In some ways it was the impact of the eccentric views of thinkers like Paracelsus (1493–1541), outraging the traditionally accepted positions, that encouraged a return to a scientific method. The basis on which the art of medicine rested, had largely remained untested and undeveloped from at least the time of Galen (AD 130–210).

7
The Theory and Practice of Tudor Medicine

Astrological and Elemental Theories

ASTROLOGICAL THEORIES

The Greek ideas of the influence of macrocosm over microcosm were still as popular as they had ever been, and even Paracelsus could not free himself from these beliefs. Platonic theories of a divinity that moves our ends had found a sympathetic chord in the mysticism of the Church. Spheres of influence which increased in perfection and potency with their distance from a geocentric earth, had recognisable spatial characteristics with a Christian heaven. The Church as a political body had no interest in dis-

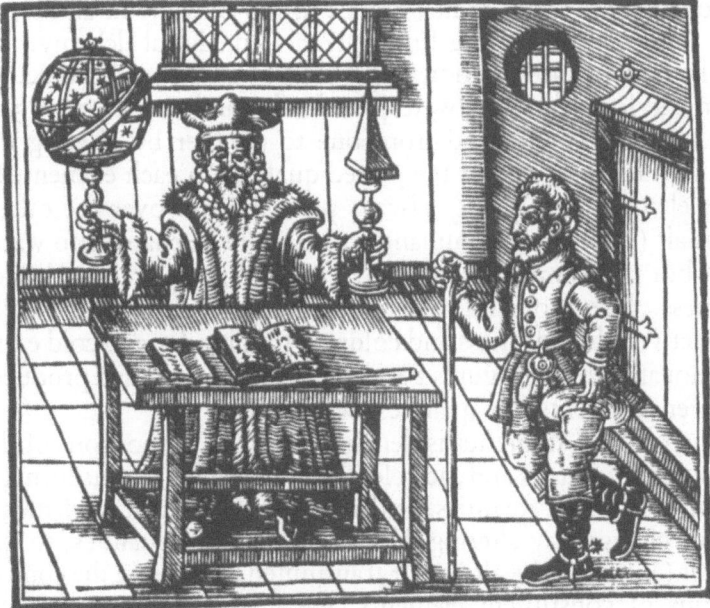

1. The title page of *The Figure-Caster or Astrologer,* 1620 edition, by John Melton.
By courtesy of the Bodleian Library.

couraging belief in the influence of things above on things below. Saint Augustine had felt it necessary to divide factual astronomy from mythical astrology, but this view never achieved popular assent. Too many astrological practitioners had a considerable vested interest in the continuance of their craft to encourage this approach (figure 1).

The theory of microcosm and macrocosm demonstrating the influence of the heavens on corresponding human parts, had been developed from Platonic ideas. The origins of astrology and the signs of the zodiac were of far greater antiquity, probably originating with the Chaldean priesthood of the Babylonians. Their interest in astronomy was determined by the desire for predictions of national and regal destiny, based on their supposed relationships to eclipses of the sun and moon. There was a need to concentrate on the ecliptic path. It is only when the moon is at or near this line of the great circle of the celestial sphere, forming the apparent orbit of the sun, that the eclipses in which they were interested can occur. In the night heavens, they noted the planets and plotted their movements among the fixed stars that lay on either side of this path. The limits of their movements defined the broader path through which the sun passes month by month. They divided this into 12 sections in relation to the 12 constellations, which are the traditional zones of the zodiac belt.

THE FOUR ELEMENTS

In this way prognosis became confused with prophecy. This accepted picture fitted the humoral theory as developed by Galen, so that movement of the bodily humours (col. pl. XX) was linked with the movement of the heavenly bodies. On this a man's health appeared to depend. Alchemy was linked with astrology in the subordination of individual metals to the sun, moon and stars. The elemental theory was fundamental to medieval alchemy.

The four qualities of hot, dry, cold and wet were combined to form the four elements water, earth, fire and air (see page 37). These could be changed from one to another by altering the predominance of one of the paired qualities in each element. In each element one quality always predominates over the other. Thus air (hot but predominantly wet) could be changed to water (wet but predominantly cold) by virtue of the shared quality of wetness. Fire (hot and dry) plus water (wet and cold) could respectively lose dryness and coldness to form dry and cold earth and hot and wet air (figures 2 and 3). The form alters and produces different elements; the qualities are basic.

The form of all matter is dependent on the proportions of the elements it contains and each element is dependent for its form on a combination of qualities. It therefore follows that as elements can be changed by altering the combinations of qualities, so can metals (as matter) be altered or transmuted by altering the combinations of constituent elements. It can thus be seen that the

48

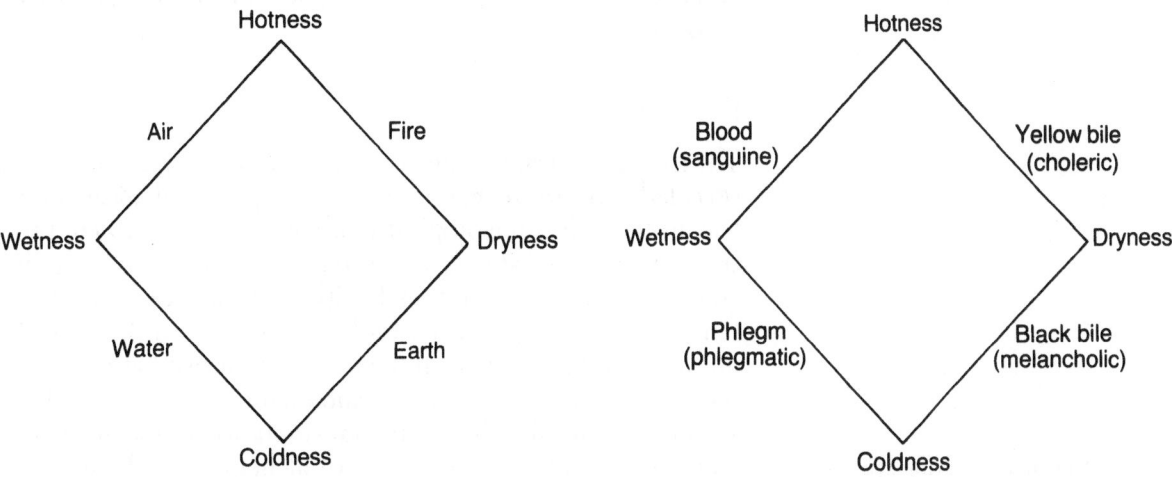

2. The four qualities and elements.

3. The four qualities, humours and tempers.

fundamental thinking was still that of the Greeks although it was embellished and often corrupted by the more confused interpretations of the later practitioners.

The four galenical humours, yellow bile, black bile, blood and phlegm which also shared the paired qualities, required that a predominantly moist disease had to be treated by a dry remedy, while a cold medicine served against a hot disease. This was known as the doctrine of contraries and its drugs as galenicals. Its practitioners required to know the imbalance of humours relating to particular diseases and the qualities to be found in the herbs, so that they could choose appropriate contraries. Herbs, like metals were subject to astrological influences.

Astrological and alchemical ideas appealed particularly to the Arabs, whose influence reinforced their acceptance in Europe. Although Copernicus (1473–1543) was to demonstrate that the whole of geocentric astronomy was based on a false assumption, and the planets and stars were not in the positions assigned by their astrological roles, neither he nor Galileo (1564–1642) achieved any more of an adverse effect on astrology than had Saint Augustine. Astrology had been based on a calculated observation, and like alchemy had been easily linked with the current religious philosophy, which ensured its survival long after improved methods of scientific observation had proved the unreliability of the precepts on which it rested. As late as 1652, Elias Ashmole's *Theatricum Chemicum Botanicum* contains the alchemical horoscopes from Thomas Norton's *Ordinall of Alchimy,* and there were others afterward. It was therefore to be expected that lesser men before them should also use a practice of great antiquity and continuing respectability.

Natural magic was another force that still had to be contended with. The supernatural produced abnormalities that required appropriate incantations, amulets and the like for prophylaxis and treatment. The Church, itself, was not averse to miraculous healing. The earlier philosophers of the Middle Ages had disputed much of the fantasy which many educated men of Tudor times accepted. A contemporary diagnostician had to take this into account.

Paracelsus

The mystic experimentalism of alchemy, although its medical arm revealed a desire to break away from post-Galenical tradition, was itself no less teleologically orientated. It was to fall short of success by its weakness of setting and seeking an unattainable goal. Transmutation of metals ultimately was dependent on the same theory that governed traditional Galenical thought. Technological improvements in the processes of distillation, crystallisation, calcination, fusion and sublimation were achieved by the alchemists, but the aim of the transmutation of metals frustrated real breakthrough. The essence of alchemy was the determined search in alchemical laboratories for the philosopher's stone, sometimes referred to as the Elixir of Life. Not only was this believed to have the power of changing base into precious metals, but when found would also have the property of conferring eternal human life. The thinking in support of such changes of

4. Paracelsus, line engraving 1540.
   By courtesy of the Royal College of Physicians, London.

5. Thomas Linacre (1466–1524).
   By courtesy of the Royal College of Physicians, London.

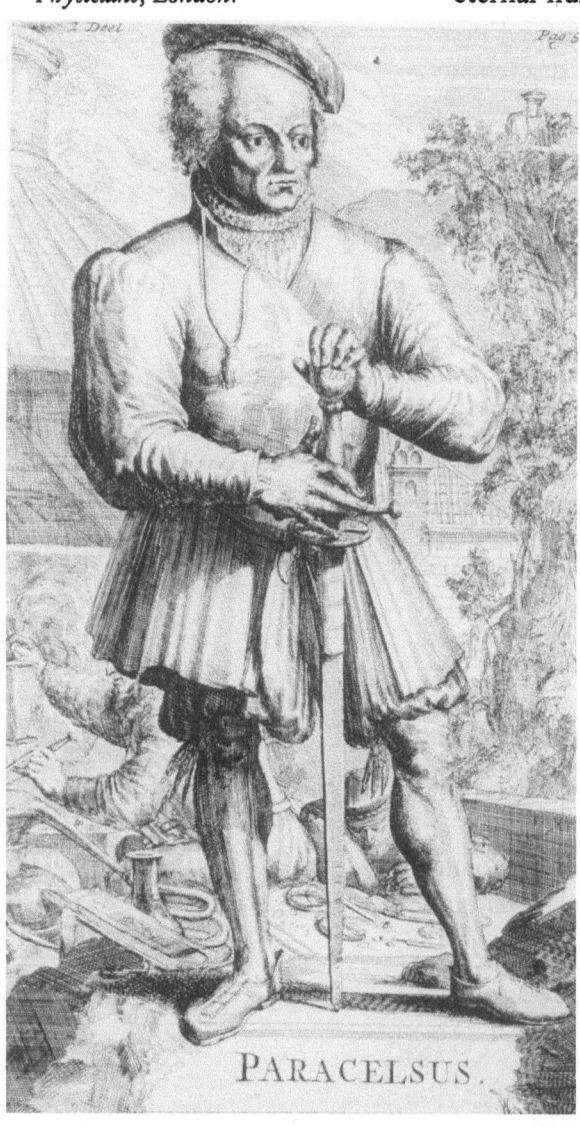

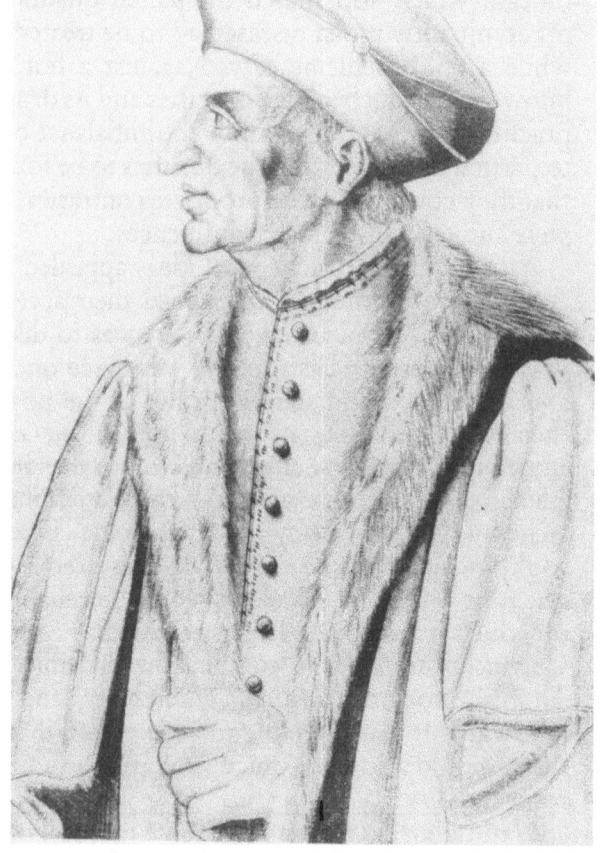

state, was parallel to that of the power of prayer to change the basic sinfulness of man to the state of perfection attainable through divine grace.

Paracelsus (figure 4) had an alchemical background from his father and from Sigismund Fugger, his employer in the Tyrolean mines where he studied metals after his student days at Basle. His was a complex character. Vituperative against his contemporaries, and their prophet Galen; eccentric and revolutionary in his practice and uncouth in his manner and dress, he was unloved by the profession. Because of his pompous personality he had relentlessly denied the skills of his contemporaries, and the Galenical theories and simple herbal remedies on which they relied for treatment. He was content with nothing, not even his already grandiose name Theóphrastus Bombastus von Hohenheim, for to this he added Paracelsus – equal to Celsus – and then again Philippus Aureolus for good measure.

Paracelsus was concerned with the application of alchemical theory to the hidden powers of medicines, his *arcana*, in restoring sickness to health in like manner of base metal to gold. He was particularly interested in the therapeutic potentialities of the metals with which he worked. The metal was but the medium of the spiritual power hidden within it. No less mystical was his revival of the 'doctrine of signatures'. Remedies could be recognised by their likeness to the disease, such as yellow celandine for jaundice. They had been deliberately made so by Divine Providence to indicate their value.

Galen

Galen's works held pride of place among the medical texts available in Britain. His teleological views were acceptable to the church, and as ill-luck would have it, to the detriment of much of his scientific work. No young doctor for generations to come was inspired to continue his initial demonstrations. Instead, the emphasis was on the humoral theory and unfortunately also on his erroneous views of the venous and arterial systems, which flourished fortuitously because of their insistence on the vital spirit, natural spirit and animal spirit. These 'spiritual' undertones captured the popular imagination to the exclusion of his sounder physiological work on the nervous system. In anatomy, his dissections of the barbary ape showed the muscles and he also wrote a book on bones for beginners. Above all else, in Tudor times, he was thought of as the 'prince of physicians' and collected editions of his clinical works were much in demand. His book on morbid swellings was available in English translation from 1586 onward. Medical scholars such as Linacre devoted themselves to Latin translations of Galen's works in an attempt to provide new and more accurate vistas of Greek medical knowledge. Such pedantic devotion encouraged attention to the form and meaning of the content rather than a desire to search nature for truth, as Galen had done. When nature was looked at in the sixteenth century it was done only to prove the correctness of Galen's teaching rather than to improve and enlarge on his pioneering work (col. pl. XXI).

Galen was infinitely more popular with the Tudor physician as a clinical writer than was Hippocrates. His case histories, larded with philosophy were far woollier than the signs and symptoms, succinctly described, listed and grouped with prognostic significance as classically taught to show the Hippocratic principles. In the Hippocratic writings one feels the importance given to clinical observation as a guide to prognosis. The treatise on Ancient Medicine in the Hippocratic Corpus, even inveighs against the theory of the four qualities as unsubstantiated and decries those who rely on theories in medicine. Galen who acknowledged Hippocrates as master, takes a more anecdotal air, as exemplified in his story of his cure of Marcus Aurelius. One feels that the message Galen wishes to deliver concerns his cure of the emperor.

THE CURE OF MARCUS AURELIUS

He begins his account with self praise, 'What happened in the case of the emperor himself was really wonderful'. All the physicians of his entourage had diagnosed his indisposition as caused by the onset of fever. After several days of ineffectual treatment Galen was summoned to the palace. He stood by silent, while the other doctors continued to feel his pulse. The emperor rather irritably asked why Galen did not bother to do so. Galen replied that the other two gentlemen who were doing this already had the benefit of knowing its norm, as they had had previous experience of its nature. The emperor then somewhat more testily told him he had better get on with his examination, which was the opportunity for which Galen had been waiting. He took the pulse and, taking his age and constitution into account, decided that this betokened no onset of fever, but rather that the stomach was overloaded with the food he had taken, which had 'turned to phlegm'.

Galen asserts that this diagnosis seemed praiseworthy to the emperor who exclaimed, 'That's it. I feel it myself. It's exactly what you say. I've taken too much cold food'. He then asked him what was to be done, and had the reply, 'If it were anyone else in this state, I should follow my custom and give him wine sprinkled with pepper. But in the case of kings like yourself, physicians are in the habit of giving safer remedies; hence it will be enough to apply over your stomach some wool impregnated with warm spikenard ointment'. Now, as Galen undoubtedly had suspected, this was what the emperor always used to do, although he invariably used purple wool for added regality. So, ordering his attendant to follow the usual custom, he dismissed Galen. The account concludes, 'When this application had been made, and his feet thoroughly heated by rubbing with a warm hand, he asked for some Sabine wine, sprinkled pepper in it, and drank'. After this cure, no praise was too great for Galen, and he adds, 'Further, as you know, he keeps constantly saying about me that I am "First among the physicians and alone among the philosophers" '.

GREEK AND ARABIC TEXTS

The Arabs loved a good story, and it was fortunate that they liked those of Galen, so that this compiler of much of the best in Greek medicine had his works preserved by them for the ultimate benefit of Western Europe. By this time, in England, Greek texts had been available for some time from Arab sources, through which medium they had survived the centuries of the Dark Ages. Translation and retranslation by Syrians, Persians and Jews had corrupted the original texts, but they still had a great following. The Europeans who belonged to the school that favoured Arabic texts were known as Arabists. The Renaissance, with its literary revival of the Greek and Roman classics, brought the desire for purer texts. These people were encouraged by the appearance at Milan in 1443 of the *De Medicina* of Celsus which had remained unheard of for centuries by Arabs and the Western World. Those like Caius and Linacre (figure 5), who preferred a return to the original writers of the humanities, were known as Humanists. Preoccupation with the literary merits was not calculated to advance the cause of science, but it must not be supposed that the protagonists in this wordy battle were not concerned with the practice of medicine. Perhaps such controversies as whether bleeding was better performed on the same side as the lesion, proximal to it, or on the opposite side and distal, which separated the derivationists of the Humanist school from the revulsionists of the Arabic school, became irrelevant when Harvey discovered that the blood circulated. As is the way with such things, it then excited much bitterness.

8
The Stuarts

Medical Advances under the Stuarts

The reign of the Tudors came to an end with Elizabeth I's death in 1603, when the Stuart King James VI of Scotland became James I of England. The Stuart period was to see the beginnings of modern descriptive medicine; numeration and experiment were called upon to become the supporters of theory, and medical science was reborn. This did not mean that enlightenment spread through the ranks of all medical practitioners. Many preferred to continue with the traditional humoral and galenic practice. Conservatism in the medical profession has always been strong. The first rays of a new understanding were just discernible, and henceforth it would be easier for a scientific view to be taken of disease and its treatment.

WILLIAM HARVEY (1578–1657)

The demonstration of the circulation of the blood, published in Stuart times in William Harvey's *De Motu Cordis* (1628) (col. pl. XXII), was of prime importance because it successfully related theory to experimental proof. It diminished the awe held for the purely metaphysical approach to medical theory, based on hypo-

1. The title page of Thomas Sydenham's *The Complete Method of Curing Almost All Diseases*, 1694 edition. *By courtesy of the Royal College of Physicians, London.*

2. The Cripplegate burial register, 1665. *Reproduced by permission of The Bodley Head from Bell's* The Great Plague.

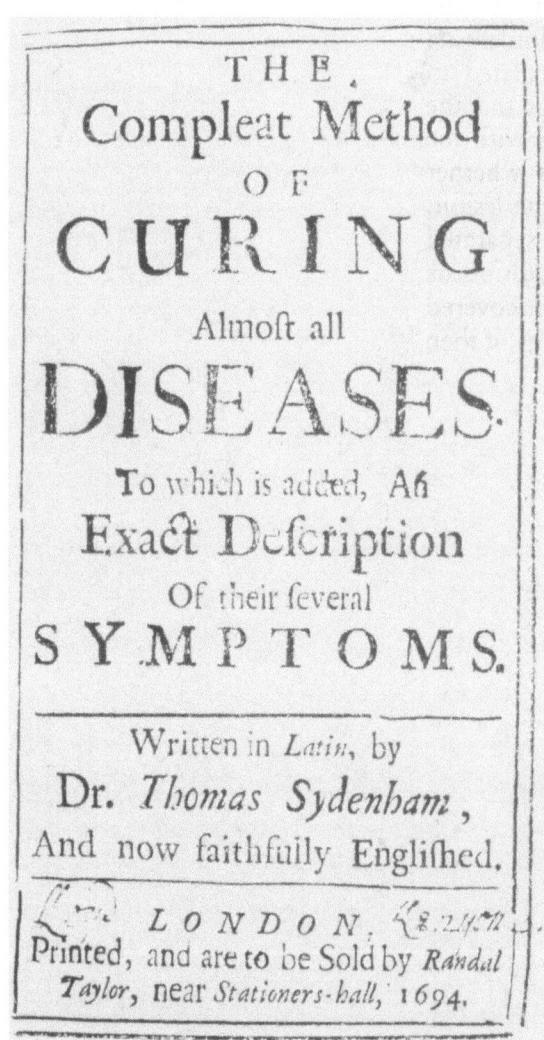

THE
Compleat Method
OF
CURING
Almoſt all
DISEASES.
To which is added, An
Exact Deſcription
Of their ſeveral
SYMPTOMS.

Written in *Latin*, by
Dr. *Thomas Sydenham*,
And now faithfully Engliſhed.

LONDON,
Printed, and are to be Sold by *Randal Taylor*, near *Stationers-hall*, 1694.

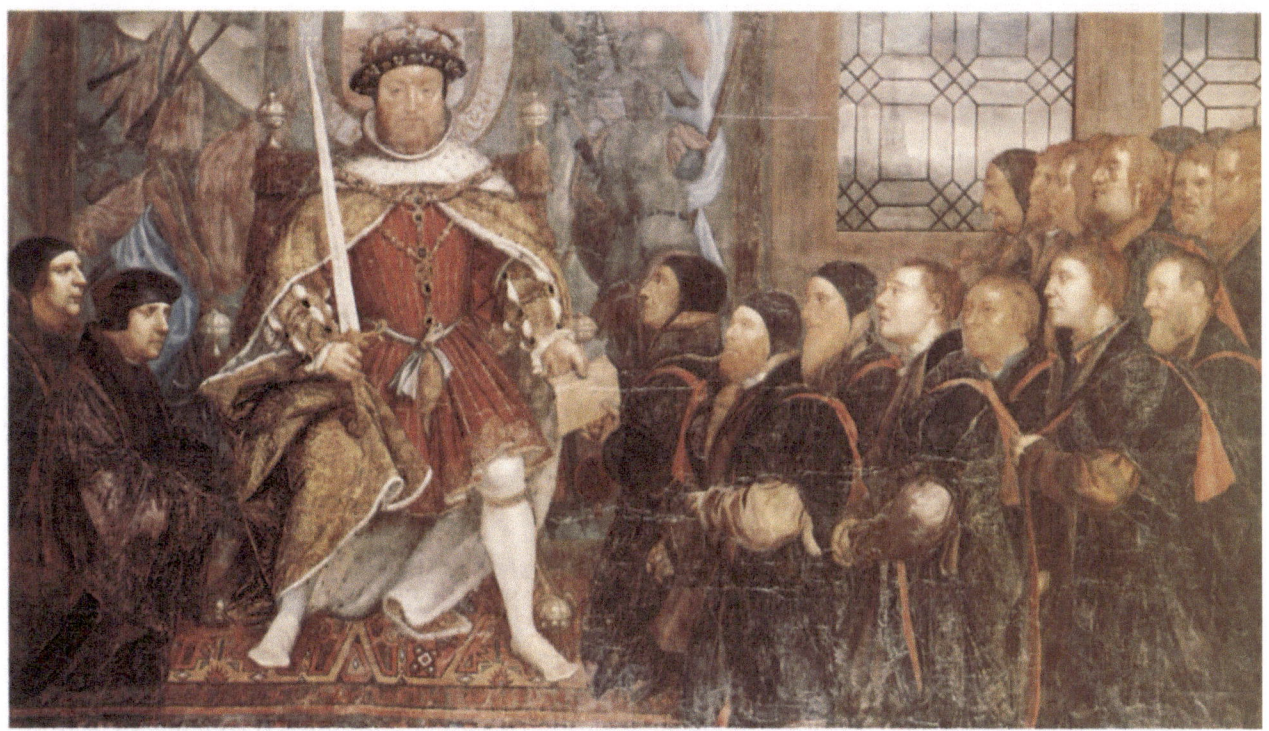

XVIII
Henry VIII and the
Barber-Surgeons, by Holbein.
*By kind permission of the
President and Council of the
Royal College of Surgeons of
England.*

XIX
John Banester delivering a
visceral lecture at the
Barber-Surgeons' Hall, London,
1581. From Hunter MS 364,
John Banester's *Anatomical
Tables.*
*By courtesy of Glasgow
University Library.*

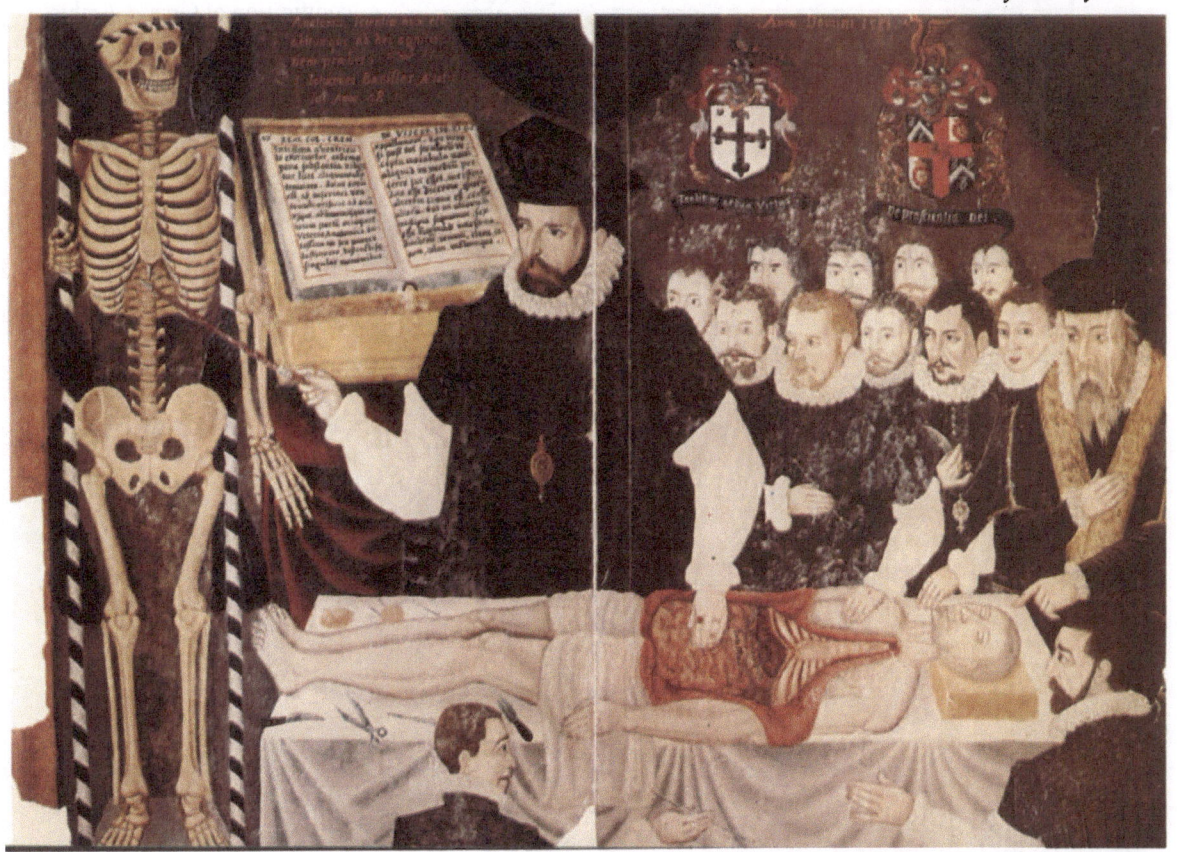

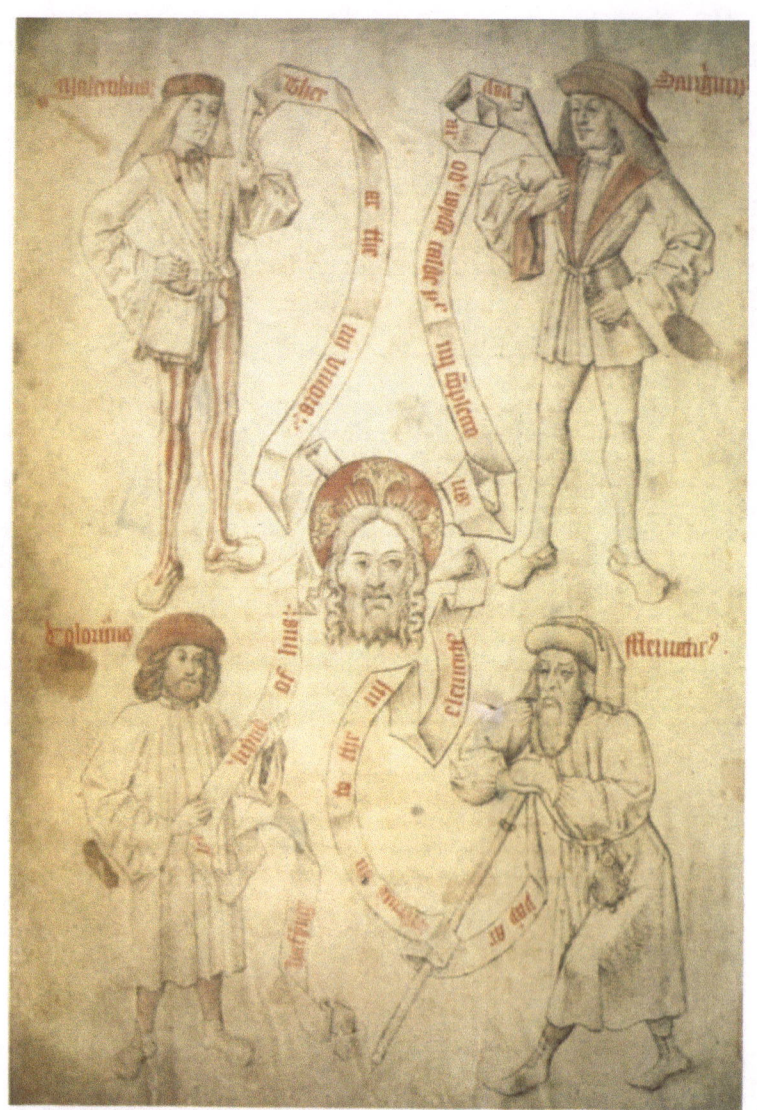

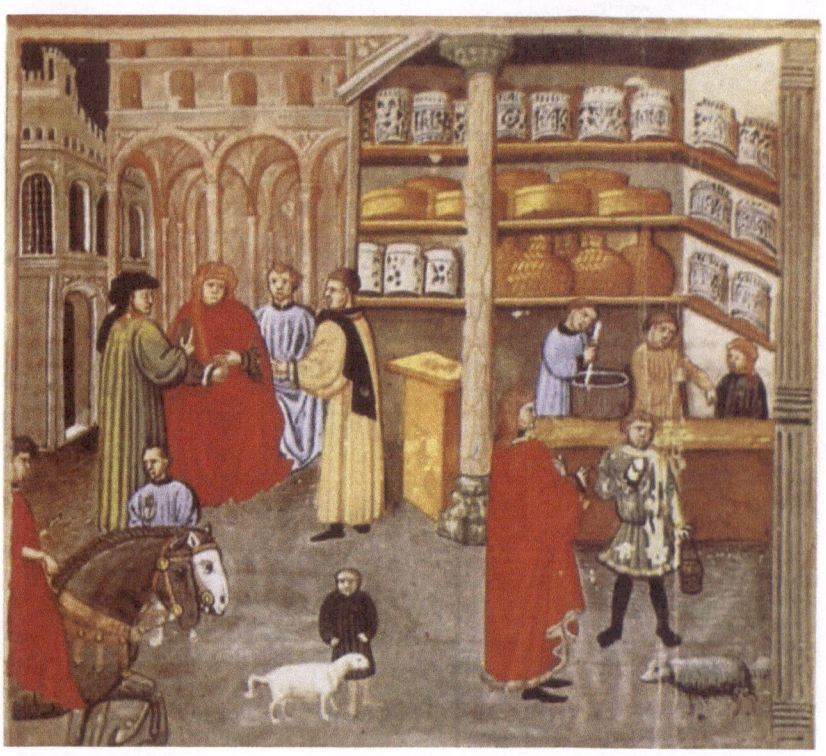

thesis and on syllogism alone. It was not abstract argument, but reasoning supported by experimental proof and as such the foundation of a physiological approach to medicine. Yet his medical practice was disappointingly galenical. He does not even seem to have utilised his 'minute-watch', which he used in his cardiac experiments, to count the pulse of patients. Neither did he avail himself of Sanctorius Sanctorius' clinical thermometer (1625), preferring to estimate fever by application of his hand. In dealing with patients, he found it comforting to retain a belief in the humoral theories and he continued to recommend venesection, 'For daily experience satisfies us that blood letting has a most salutary effect in many diseases, and is indeed the foremost among all the general remedial means'. In his dealings with patients, the rationalist could not abandon empiricism. Empiricism comforts the bodily physician when, aware of the shortcomings of science, he still has occasion to rely on traditional remedies.

His prescriptions also illustrate his humoral beliefs, although they are simpler than those written by most of his contemporaries. Dr Gweneth Whitteridge has transcribed and annotated one of Harvey's prescriptions for John Aubrey in 1653:

Px fol. sennae 3 fs.
    Rhubarbari, Agarici,
    Radicis Hellebori nigri,
    Seminarum anisi,
        feoniculi, ana 3 i.
    liquoris hissopi magistralis 3 i fs.
    passularum P. i.
    Fiat decoctio in aquae et vini albi ana q.s. ad colaturae
    3 iiij fs.
    Adde syrupi magistralis purgantis ad Melancholiam,
        syrupi rosacei solutivi, ana 3 i.
        aquae cinnamomi guttae vj.
    Misce.
    Capiat cum custodia.
    Postera die emittatur sanguis ex vena hepatica dextri
    brachii ad 3 ij.

This purgative mixture contained rhubarb and syrup of roses to treat the excess of yellow bile, senna and hellebore against the black bile and agaric against phlegm. The aniseed and fennel were to cure flatulence. The P stands for 'pugillus' meaning a 'pinch', and the substance 'passula' could be either raisins or prunes.

Not surprisingly, John Aubrey commented that Harvey's prescriptions were not highly regarded by his colleagues. Indeed, Richard Glover, the apothecary at St Bartholomew's Hospital once claimed that Harvey had killed a patient with an overdose of colocynth. He was exonerated on the grounds that the apothecary had not shown him the prescription, a defence that would have a sympathetic hearing today.

THOMAS SYDENHAM (1624–1689)

There were physicians such as Thomas Sydenham (pl. XXIII), who, whilst guiding clinical practice to some considerable advancement, professed an almost total disdain for theory (figure 1). Like William Harvey, Thomas Sydenham was not entirely able to free himself from the past and achieve a purity of ideal. In his clinical observations, his method was hippocratic rather than galenical: facts rather than speculation. Whereas Hippocrates was primarily interested in prognosis, Sydenham was interested in disease entities, 'It is necessary that all disease be reduced to definite and certain species, and that with the same care which we see exhibited by botanists in their phytologies'. He relied on his case-histories for building up the pattern of disease. However, he too was a humoralist, and went so far as to write an essay *Of the four constitutions*. Yet he was sufficiently free-thinking to use quinine, in the form of Peruvian bark, for intermittent fevers on a recently founded empirical basis. Of the men of this era, Thomas Sydenham emerges as the prototype of the idealised general practitioner of the next two centuries. A conscientious, conservative, almost puritanically moral doctor (he was a Puritan) with an intense desire to be a disease detective.

Medical practice had been disturbed by the recent advances, but it left the average practitioner largely unchanged. The keener ones engaged their talents in the natural sciences, but this left the conduct of their own practices almost untouched, as one can see with William Harvey and Giorgio Baglivi. Everybody, including the great innovators, were too near the new discoveries. The greatest of them were not able to appreciate the influence of each other's work, even when it impinged on their own fields.

THE DISCOVERIES OF OTHER PRACTITIONERS

The Great Systems of the seventeenth century were the hinterland between Aristotelian and modern science. The new discoveries posed problems for which the work done had not advanced enough to provide answers. René Descartes (1596–1650) tried to assemble and elaborate on this work. He used the new knowledge, such as Harvey on the circulation, and Snell on refraction, even though he understood it imperfectly, and added his own innovations to produce a new physiology. Iatrochemists, like Thomas Willis (1621–1675), who built on Cartesianism, theorised in terms of chemical changes rather than along humoral lines. Iatrophysicists of some repute, like Giorgio Baglivi (1668–1706), the Italian who distinguished smooth and striped muscle, seem to have felt that this sort of laboratory work did not help the patient. Garrison quotes him as saying, 'To frequent societies, to visit libraries, to own valuable unread books or shine in all the journals does not in the least contribute to the comfort of the sick'.

Willis, who fought on the other side from Sydenham in the Civil War, was a practising physician who observed disease, and who will forever be remembered by medical students as the man who described the sweet taste of diabetic urine. In his London *Practice of Physick* (1685) he describes myasthenia gravis. He was astute enough to note the phenomenon of paracusis in a deaf woman, who could only hear speech when a drum was beating. He also wrote his famous *Cerebri Anatome* (1664), illustrated by Sir Christopher Wren.

CLASSIFICATION OF DISEASE

The new interest in the cause and nature of disease led to the classification of diseases. The pioneer medical statistician John Graunt (1620–1674), however, had little confidence in the named causes of death, which in some places were reported by lay searchers rather than doctors, to the parish clerks. He wrote:

When anyone dies, then, either by tolling, or ringing of a bell, or by bespeaking of a grave by the sexton, the same is known to the searchers, corresponding with the said sexton. The searchers hereupon (who are antient matrons, sworn to their office) repair to the place where the dead

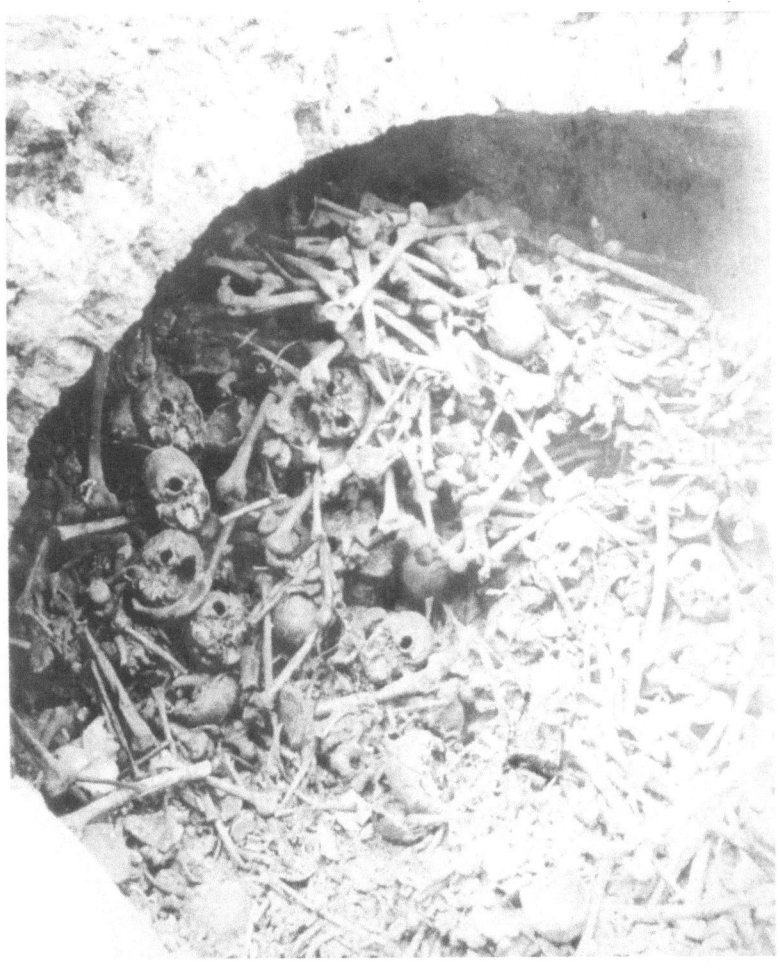

3. A burial site for plague victims in London about 1664.
   By courtesy of the Wellcome Trustees.

corps lies, and by views of the same, and by other enquiries, they examine by what disease or casualty the corps died. Hereupon they make their report to the parish clerk.

The searchers had to rely on evidence from neighbours and relatives and:

The old women searchers after the mist of a cup of ale, and the bribe of a two-groat fee, instead of one, given them, cannot tell whether this emaciation or leanness were from a phthisis or from an hectic fever, atrophy, etc.

These women could be bribed to conceal either death by violence or the plague (figures 2 and 3). The cause of death had to depend on what could be learnt from local people and a qualified physician could do no more as he could tell little from an external inspection of the dead body (figure 4).

4. The manner of dissecting the pestilential body. Frontispiece of Thomson's *Loimotomia*. *Reproduced by permission of The Bodley Head from Bell's* The Great Plague.

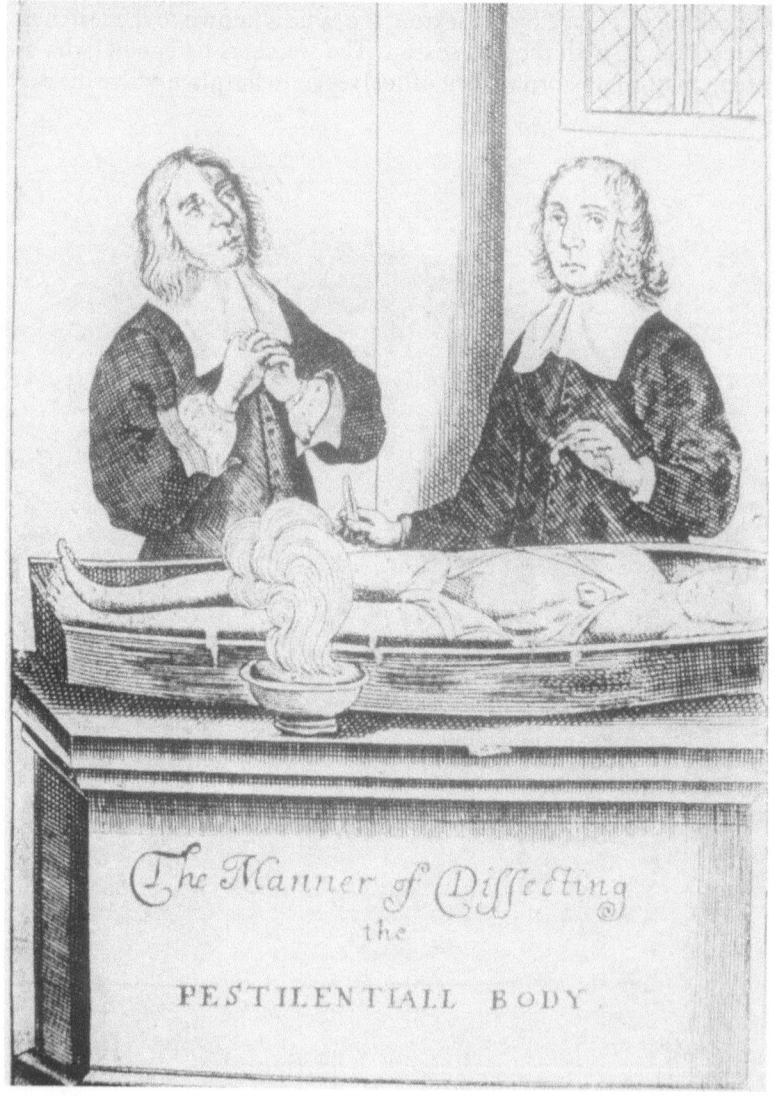

The Manner of Dissecting
the
PESTILENTIALL BODY.

THE IMPACT OF THE NEW DISCOVERIES ON MEDICAL PRACTICE

Medical science made great advances with the development of the microscope and the improvement in gross descriptive anatomy. The practitioners were also studying function. Above all, experimental proof was recognised as essential and the humoral theories and astrology no longer held pride of place in medical theory and practice.

There was no clear relationship between the discoveries of the natural scientists and the treatment of disease: the scientists themselves often seemed to find little relevance between their specialised work and their clinical practice. Their discoveries often posed problems which could not be answered, as their work was not sufficiently advanced. Therefore, although medical practice was disturbed by these advances, it is not surprising that the average practitioner, both graduate and non-graduate, did not improve his clinical practice.

In the actual day-to-day practice of medicine there was still a great deal of superstition. Many followed the astrological and alchemical ideas of Nicholas Culpeper (1616–1654), who was himself an apothecary. Sir Kenelm Digby (1603–1665), a member of the Royal Society, believed in the weapon salve, which was used to anoint the weapon which caused the wound, and not the wound itself. He also invented a Sympathetic Powder, which was the basis of his fortune. It was a century of private and secret nostrums, even William Harvey had one. The successive London Pharmacopoeias bore testimony to a faith in the efficacy of blood, fat, bile, sweat, swallows' nests and criminals' bones. The sovereign, Charles II, still touched for scrofula, known as the King's Evil (figure 5).

The Apothecaries

THE EFFECT OF THE APOTHECARIES' CHARTER

The royal apothecary Gideon de Laune (col. pl. XXIV), and the royal physician Sir Theodore de Mayerne, both of foreign birth, petitioned King James I to grant the apothecaries a royal charter (col. pl. XXV). The King consented in 1617 because he felt, 'Grocers are but merchants, the business of an apothecary is a Mistery, wherefore I think it be fitting they be a Corporation of themselves'.

In their search for professional status, the apothecaries decided, 'to put their dependence upon the liberal-minded College of Physicians'. They found that they had misplaced their confidence; no sooner had the King died than the physicians sought to dominate 'those lowly dispensers of drugs and boluses'. The physicians saw the apothecaries as a threat to their incomes. Therefore, although they were prepared to help the apothecaries gain independence and a monopoly in the sale of medicines, they stipulated that they must limit their dispensing to Collegiate physicians, who at this time numbered a mere 40 in London.

The result was a fiasco. The apothecaries faced competition from both the grocers, who continued to sell spices, and the non-Collegiate physicians and surgeons, who were now forced to do their own dispensing. The apothecaries, therefore, had achieved their ambition of independence but at a cost to their livelihood and their rights as ordinary citizens of London. Their wits had been sharpened by these threats to their livelihood proving that wealth has always been of more immediate significance than status, for Cecil had said, gentility, is 'nought else but old riches'.

THE DECLINE IN THE PHYSICIANS' POWER

Raach's *Directory of English Country Physicians 1603-1643* shows that a relatively large number of medical practitioners received a university education. He lists 814 doctors, of which 635 had matriculated at a university, mostly Oxford and Cambridge, and 137 had attended the continental universities, of Padua, Leyden, Basle, Caen, Montpellier and Rheims. Out of a total of 246 MDs, 75 were gained on the continent. They practised medicine throughout England, in large towns, villages and hamlets, and they prospered. The home counties and the coast attracted a large proportion, for they were the most heavily populated. During this period Norwich had 17, Canterbury 22, Exeter 13 and York 10, and Ramsbury, Wiltshire, Weston sub Edge, Gloucestershire and Bradhembury, Devon, could also boast their own medical practitioners.

THE RISE OF THE APOTHECARIES

The Civil War interfered with the established balances of power. Outbreaks of plague in London moved the physicians out of town more readily than the apothecaries. By the time the countryside had settled down after the Restoration, traditional privileges had been undermined. On their return to London, the physicians found that the apothecaries and surgeons were more numerous and more widely active in practice. They tried to undermine the apothecaries' trade by setting up their own public dispensary at the College in 1696, supplying medicines at cost, and more dispensaries followed, but they were unprofitable. The merchant class preferred to seek the personal attention of an apothecary rather than visit a public dispensary.

It was the time of the pamphlet war between the apothecaries and physicians, another indication of the insecurity of the physicians who no longer felt that they could rely on privilege to maintain their position in the hierarchy of medicine. In the seventeenth century, as a result of the upheavals in medical theory and changes in civic structure, the position of the apothecary as the man in his shop, who could provide a diagnosis, dispense his own prescription, dress wounds and even bleed without the help of either physician or surgeon, made him the most easily available

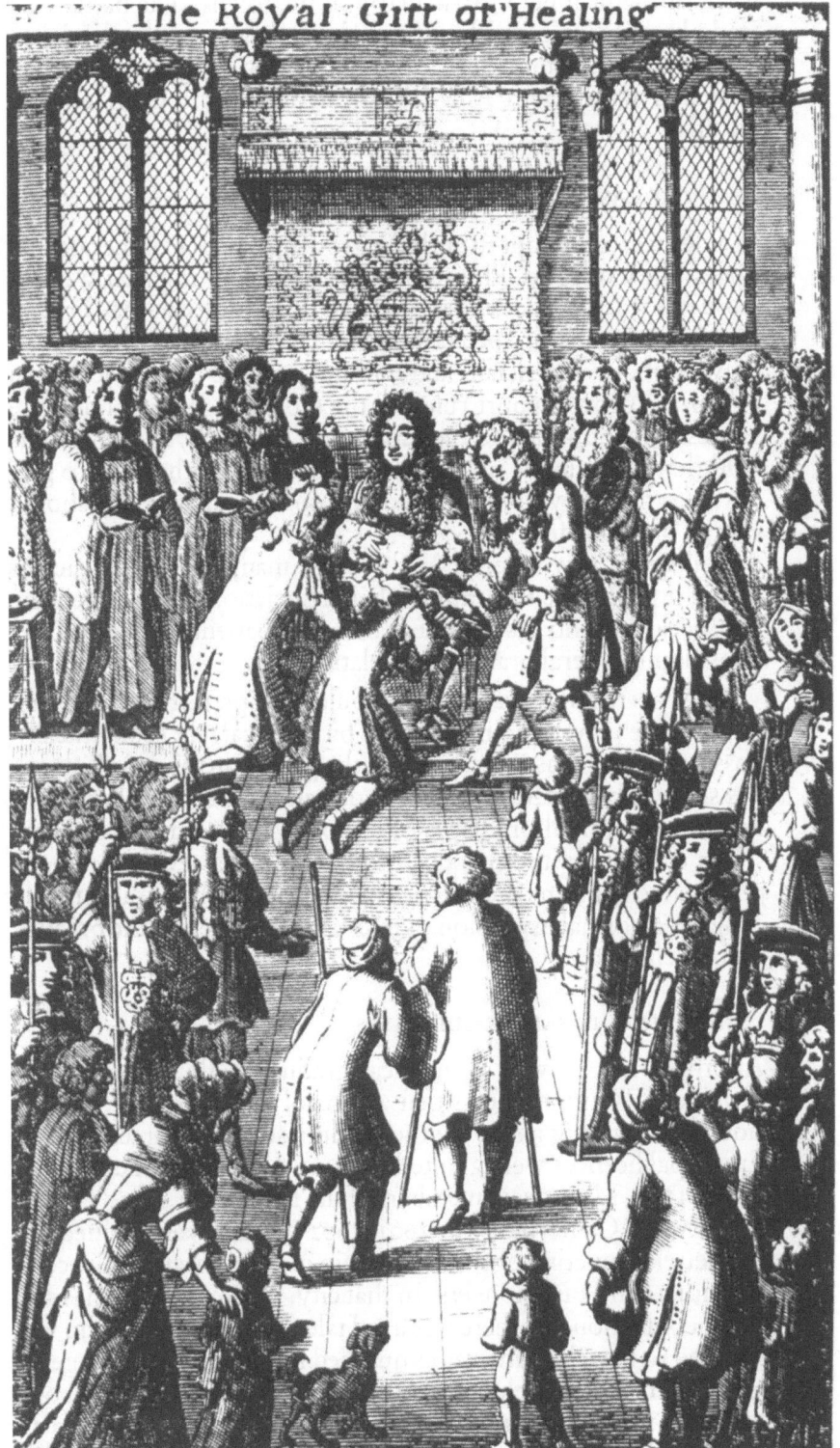

The Royal Gift of Healing

form of medical help, particularly in the towns. The battle over trade had emancipated him from dependence on the physician. His financial strengthening, by the opening drug trade with the East and with South America, brought him the confidence of wealth.

THE ROSE CASE

In a desperate attempt to curb the growing practice of the apothecaries, the College of Physicians took legal action against William Rose in 1703. The College alleged that this apothecary had broken the Act of 1523 in prescribing for John Seale, 'without the Advice of any Physician, and without any Fee for Advice taken by him'. A lower court ruled in the College's favour, but Rose successfully appealed to the House of Lords in 1703. The Lords held that it was in the public interest to allow apothecaries to give advice when they compounded and sold medicines but should charge only one fee.

Following this reversal in fortunes, many of the physicians found it profitable to continue their associations with dispensing apothecaries who also looked after the patients, developing a consultant-general practitioner relationship.

There were apothecaries who would have preferred to concentrate on the practice of medicine. This was scarcely economically possible, being frustrated both by the physicians and, as Roberts has shown, by the Society of Apothecaries itself. Members were denied the normal privileges of seniority if they devoted themselves entirely to the practice of physic. It was evidently more practical to combine the practice of medicine with the sale of their drugs as a normal expansion of trade, than to attempt the practice of medicine alone.

LINKS WITH THE BARBER-SURGEONS

Apothecaries, as well as medical graduates, flourished in the provinces. Whittet reports that at Bristol they were men of considerable standing and were the wealthiest general practitioners. Episcopal licences were granted to them, for Edward Tucker had one in 1672. Many were members of the Barber-Surgeons' Gild of the city. In Canterbury, in 1601–1602 decrees were ratified for the better regulating of the Fellowship of Apothecaries, Grocers, Chandlers and Fishmongers. In that city, where apothecaries still made confectionery, there was a sad tale of an apprentice who was allowed to have his indentures quashed following brutal usage by his master, which included chastisement over the use of a wrong mould in making a marchpane for an alderman's christening party (c 1610). In Coventry, too, the apothecaries were strengthening their links with the barber-surgeons. In 1673 they agreed 'That the apothecaryes and Barber-Chirurgeons were to be an incorporate company as formerly . . .' Thomas Pidgeon, apothecary, was mayor there in 1661. In Shrewsbury the apothecaries became united with the barber-surgeons in 1662, and this seems to have been the pattern elsewhere. It was more than the chance association which so often produced strange mixtures of trades and gilds. The bond was the common link of general medical practice.

The Barber-Surgeons

THE CHARTER

The Barber-Surgeons' Company continued its system of apprenticeship followed by examination. In 1629, Charles I granted the barber-surgeons a charter which enacted that:

No-one whatever should exercise for profit the science or art of Surgery in London and Westminster, or seven miles of them, until he had passed an examination . . . persons so examined might use the art in any place in the kingdom of England.

The barber-surgeons attempted to gain statutory authority for this in 1689. Their petition failed, however, because they also wanted to 'give all sorts of medicine' and the College of Physicians was still powerful enough to object successfully to this.

SURGICAL TEXTS

Richard Wiseman (1622–1676) was the surgical counterpart of Thomas Sydenham. He was a skilful and thoughtful surgeon who wrote *Severall Chiurgicall Treatises* in 1676. In 1633, Stephen Bradwell published a book on first aid called *Helps for suddain accidents endangering life*.

Licences

The bishops continued to grant licences to practise surgery, while the College of Physicians granted licences for medicine (see page 43). The University of Oxford also issued licences for medicine, '*ad practicandum in re medica per totam Angliam*'. This was given to men who had practised physic for many years, but it was also given to students of medicine, and those who already had the MD. In 1599, the University laid down certain conditions for its award: a fixed period of study, attendance at lectures and most importantly, the approval of the regius professor of medicine. On 27 June, 1614 'Richard Berry MA, Linc, was fit for MB and for lic. to pract. med.'.

The University also issued licences for surgery, '*ad practicandum in chirurgia per universam Angliam*', but these were less popular. Professor Thomas Clayton issued a licence for surgery to Bernard Wright on 30 June 1618, after ascertaining his proficiency 'by many conferences; meeting at many patients, where he hath shewed good skill, rare judgement, and dexterity: as also by his dissection of many bodies for anatomy'.

9
The House of Hanover

The Apothecaries under the House of Hanover

THE DEVELOPMENT OF MEDICAL APOTHECARIES

The ruling by the House of Lords in favour of John Rose in 1703 (see page 62), meant that apothecaries could now legally practise medicine provided they always took care not to charge for their advice in addition to the charge for the medicine. This simply meant that they were always careful to prescribe a bottle of medicine at every consultation.

The Society of Apothecaries continued to maintain its high standards for those apothecaries now practising medicine. Apprentices in England, Wales, Ireland and Scotland were examined and approved after having been bound for seven years. By 1774, there were sufficient apothecaries inside the Society engaged in the practice of medicine to allow promotion to the livery to be limited to such practising apothecaries only.

THE DEVELOPMENT OF THE CHELSEA PHYSIC GARDEN

The Society also developed its pharmaceutical side during this period. The methods of treatment were changing in response to the activities of the scientists. There was a new interest in physic gardens, imported herbs and laboratories. The laboratory, established in 1623, was concerned with making vegetable remedies, and in 1671 another had been set up to make chemical ones.

The Chelsea Physic Garden founded in 1673 (col. pl. XXVI), was held on lease and thus any improvements made by the apothecaries would benefit only the landlord after their lease had expired. In 1772, this was remedied by Sir Hans Sloane who generously acquired the garden for the apothecaries so that they could 'hold the same for ever' enabling them to distinguish the 'useful plants' from those 'that are hurtful'. He was shrewd enough to ensure that the garden was maintained as a scientific enterprise, for as such it was extremely valuable in educating the members of the Society and in encouraging botanical research.

THE RELATIONSHIP BETWEEN THE APOTHECARIES AND PHYSICIANS

Relationships between apothecaries and physicians were improving as they recognised the mutual advantages that could be gained. Sir Hans Sloane who had trained in physic at the Apothecaries Hall, later became President of the Royal College of Physicians. Nevertheless, the apothecaries remained very much a part of the City, with their roots in trade, while the physicians continued to claim the special privileges of rank and education.

The Barber-Surgeons

UNIFICATION OF THE BARBERS AND SURGEONS

The barbers and surgeons had been united into one company by the Act of 1540. The surgeons were at first delighted with the privileges they had won by joining the barbers, who were numerically far greater and consequently more powerful.

THE BARBERS

Despite the Act of 1540, the barbers and surgeons still behaved independently of each other. The barbers were precluded from active surgery within the Company by the 1540 Act:

for as muche as suche persones being the misterie or facultee of surgery, oftentymes medle and take into their cure and houses suche sicke and diseased persons as ben infected with the pestilence great pockes & such other contagious infirmityes do use or exercise barbari, as washynge, or shavyng, and other feates therunto belongyng, which is veraie perillous for infectyng the kyngs liege people resortyng to their shoppes and houses ther beyng washed or shaven.

Any barber who defied this ruling was prosecuted:

6th May, 1712. Ordered that Mr Watts be summoned to appear before the Governors att the next Court to answer a Complaint agt him for practiceing Surgery & Instructing Barbers for 2 Guineas a peice. Ordered that Mr Small be likewise summoned to appeare before the Governors att the next Court to answer a Complaint agt him for amputateing a Breast without calling an examiner to be present.

In October 1638, Thomas Bowden was fined 40s for not presenting his patient Godfrey Lee to the Company for a proper consultation, for the unfortunate Lee had died under his treatment. A further fine was imposed in that:

Being not an approved Surgian for that he tooke upon him the cure & charge of ye said Godfrey being daungerouslie wounded & did not joyne an able & approved surgian with him in that cure . . . alsoe it is ordered that for his the said Thomas Bowdens evill practise in Surgerye he shalbe Comitted to the Compter in Wood Streete.

This proved to be only a temporary setback for Thomas Bowden, however, as he was elected Third Warden in 1654 and Upper Warden in 1660.

THE SURGEONS

The bishops still issued licences to practise surgery, and continued negligent in their duties, even in the eighteenth century. As late as 1710, the Archbishop of Canterbury, through his officers, was licensing surgeons without the proper prior examination by four of their peers, as required under the Act of 1511 (see page 42). His Grace was accordingly petitioned 'not to license any person within his Diocess who hath not first obtained a Testimoniall under the Seale of our Company certifying the examination of such person & his skill & ability for the exercise of that art'. The Bishop of London was also continually in trouble over his negligent licensing.

Some Company examiners were guilty of corruption for in 1709 it had been ordered that:

No Examiner in Surgery should in future accept any gratuity from, or be treated or entertained in any manner by, any Sea Surgeon or Surgeon's Mate, either before or after examination, under the penalty of being removed from his offices of Examiner and Assistant.

The surgeons within the Company placed more emphasis on examinations than apprenticeship, because they wished to emulate the physicians who did not have to serve apprenticeships: apprenticeship was the mark of a tradesman. It was also easier to determine failure in examination than it was to detect false indentures.

The entries in the examiners' book tersely gave their reasons for the rejection of certain candidates:

13th February 1712. Wm Ogilby Rejected & said very Saucily it should be the last time.

Alexr Keith Rejected because an Apothecary's Boy.

Edward Brown Rejected because a Barber.

James Erwin ffor a Mate and rejected for Sauciness to Mr. Blundell & the Court.

William Miles was recommended to the Company by Lord Torrington, but the surgeons examined him and 'seeming to know nothing of Surgery' he was rejected. An entry for the 4th April, 1729, rejects a certain Peregrine Compton because he was 'fuddled and not answering a question'.

The surgeons examined foreign applicants for their ability to speak English as well as for their skill and knowledge in Latin and surgery. The examiners' book states that 'the Court did not think it proper' to examine foreigners such as James Ripault, a Frenchman, and John Jacob Sax, a Prussian, as neither of them could speak English.

THE SPLIT BETWEEN THE BARBERS AND THE SURGEONS

Both the wealth and skill of the professional surgeons within the Company distinguished them from the barbers. The surgeons who had served in the army and navy formed their own group in the Barber-Surgeons' Company. Inside the Company, the numbers and wealth of those men who could be called professional surgeons were increasing. Men who had served in the armed forces in this capacity had always formed a special group, and graduates, or those who held university licences, had common interests. In the eighteenth century, there were no longer just the two hospitals of St. Bartholomew and St. Thomas in London to provide employment. The founding of Westminster (1719), Guy's (1725), St. George's (1733), the Middlesex (1745), and the London (1746) created the opportunities for a new class of surgeon to develop. The barbers and surgeons continued to behave independently of each other, as indeed they had done since their incorporation.

Matters were not improved by the actions of William Cheselden (1699–1752), a freeman of the Company. He was charged before the Court of Assistants with distracting students from the public anatomy dissections which the Company had arranged, by teaching anatomy himself at his nearby house. He was apparently so prompt in claiming the bodies of 'malefactors from the place of execution' for his own use, that the Company's beadles found it 'difficult to bring away the Company's bodies'. Presumably, by the time they arrived, Cheselden had already taken the best. He promised not to do it again and it is probable that he did not go back on his word as he became a member of the Court of Assistants in 1738, and the Junior Warden in 1744.

Cheselden, however, was unhappy in the Company and in 1744 he encouraged his surgeon colleagues to break away from the barbers. The barbers opposed this move realising they would lose a great deal of their revenue without the wealthy surgeons. Despite this, the surgeons succeeded in establishing their indepen-

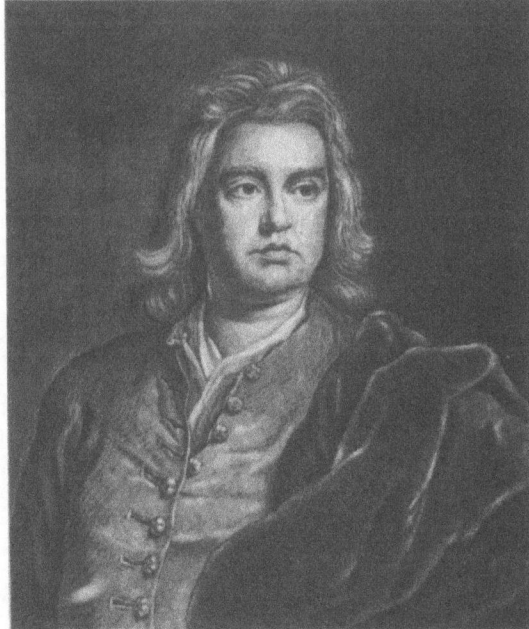

1. The trade card of Charles Peter, a surgeon.
Reproduced by permission of the Trustees of the British Museum.

67

dence once again by the Act of 1745. John Ranby, the serjeant-surgeon, was a personal friend of King George II, and as such he used his influence on the surgeons' behalf. He became the first Master of the new Surgeons' Company, followed by Cheselden in 1746.

THE SURGEONS' COMPANY

Unlike the Apothecaries' Society, the Surgeons' Company was anxious to sever its old ties with the City and commerce, and now discouraged all connections with pharmacy by prohibiting any member practising it from becoming a Court Examiner or Assistant. The new Surgeons had lost the privileges they had enjoyed as liverymen of the Barber-Surgeons' Company. Nevertheless, members of the new Company were not prevented from becoming freemen of the City of London if they so wished.

The surgeons examined all candidates before allowing them to become members of the Company, although surgeons already practising in London when the Company was formed, were allowed to join on payment of its fee, £12 14s 6d. The Company

2. The first page from George Armstrong's *Proposals for Administering Advice and Medicine to the Children of the Poor*, 1769. *By courtesy of the Wellcome Trustees.*

3. Gilray print of a country general practitioner in the eighteenth century. *By courtesy of the Royal College of General Practitioners.*

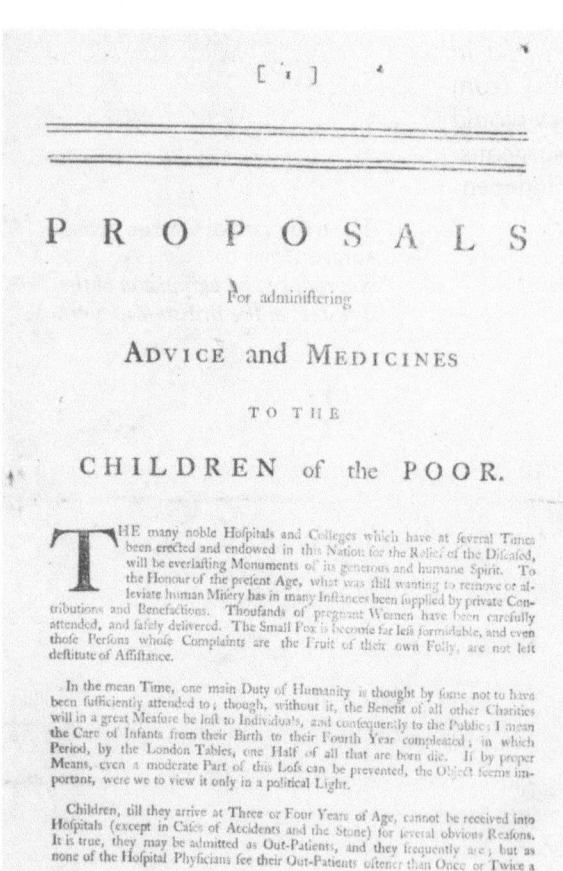

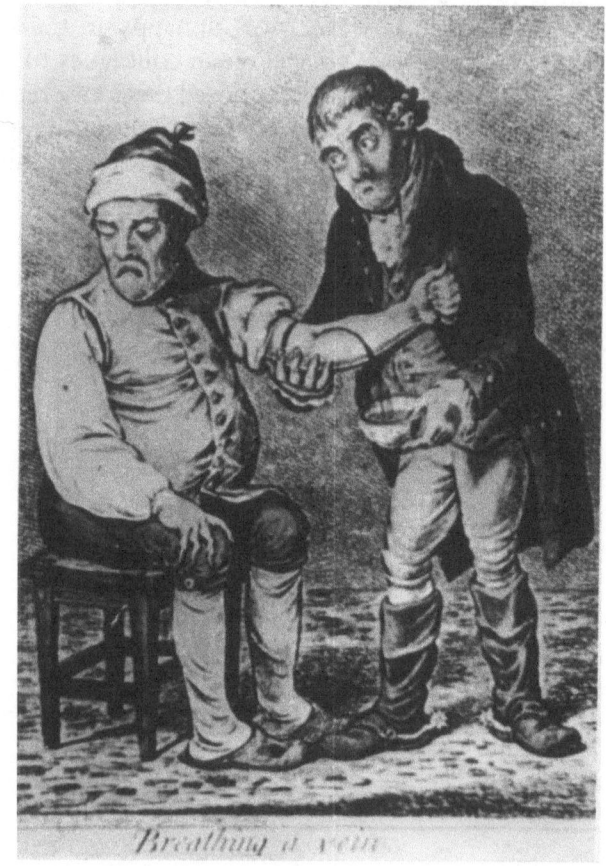

also examined surgeons who wished to serve in the army or navy, and the successful applicants were allowed to enter civilian practice at the end of a three-year period of service, without further re-examination (figure 1).

A by-law of 1748 gave control of the Company to the Court of Ten Examiners, in which the Master and two wardens were always to hold office. The examiners took the attitude that the final examination was of greater importance than the seven years' apprenticeship which the 1745 Act had enjoined. The Company's legal adviser, Thomas Erskine (1750–1823) gave it as his opinion, when consulted in 1781, that they were regulated by the Act of 1511 and not by the Statute of Apprentices. The Act of 1511, by which the Bishop of London granted a licence after examination and approval by four surgeons, does not appear to have specifically mentioned apprenticeship. However, apprenticeship persisted for a further 60 years or more despite the nonchalance of the examiners.

The entry in the *Annals of the Barber-Surgeons* concerning the medical examination for fitness of Bosun North on 14 October 1726, illustrates the day to day problems that the practitioners encountered, and how little they have changed:

Peter North Boatswain of His Majesty's ship Cornwall was viewed for superannuation and pretended to be afflicted with deafness & the Gout. But the Court being of the opinion that his deafness (if any) was occasiond by wax in his ear only, which might be cured by syringing, and not being satisfyd that he had the gout, The Court did not think fit but that he was capable of further service at Sea.

THE RELATIONSHIP BETWEEN THE SURGEONS AND PHYSICIANS

It was becoming easier to recognise grades of practitioners who had been given a clear certificate of competence as apothecaries, surgeons or physicians, though sometimes they changed their allegiance.

In 1711, a Daniell Turner paid £50 to be discharged from the Company of Barber-Surgeons so that he could become a Collegiate physician. Similarly, William Hunter wanted to leave the Company of Surgeons to become a physician, but the College would not admit him while he was still a member of the Company. He had to pay 40 guineas in order to leave the Surgeons and a further 20 guineas when they discovered that he had taken the College's licence without their permission. Later they reconsidered their decision and returned the 20 guineas to him on the grounds that he had not deliberately broken their rules but had simply omitted to inform them.

Rural Medical Practice

The work of R. S. McConaghey has provided some details about eighteenth century rural medical practice in Torrington, a town of 2,000 people. A group of unqualified women provided valuable medical care for the poor and on certain occasions their work was financially rewarded by the parish. A 'strange woman' was paid 11s for curing the leg of Richard White, and Mrs Bond of Bideford was given 5s for curing Jon Thorne of the itch. The tombstone of Prudence Potter, the wife of the rector of Newton St Petrock, a nearby village, states that she spent her life 'in the industrious, charitable and successful practice of physic, chirurgry and midwifery'.

The parish paid a Dr Craddock an annual salary of five guineas for treating the poor. There were also other regular practitioners such as Dr Bradford who received 10s for his 'cure on the mouth of Grace the wife of Thomas Dolben being fretted with a canker'. Dr Richard Chubb of Exeter specialised in eyes and in 1707 he received £5 7s 6d for 'couching a cataract in ye eye of Grace ye wife of Richard Saunders'. In 1718 he was given £2 12s 6d for treating the bad eyes of William Rook's daughter and for curing 'Thomas Riches broken leg'. The apothecary Philip Potter, who was the great-uncle of Joshua Reynolds, received £7 10s in 1707 for physic for poor people (figures 2 and 3).

4. 'The Doctor's Visit' (1720–1725) by William Hogarth.
By courtesy of the Tate Gallery.

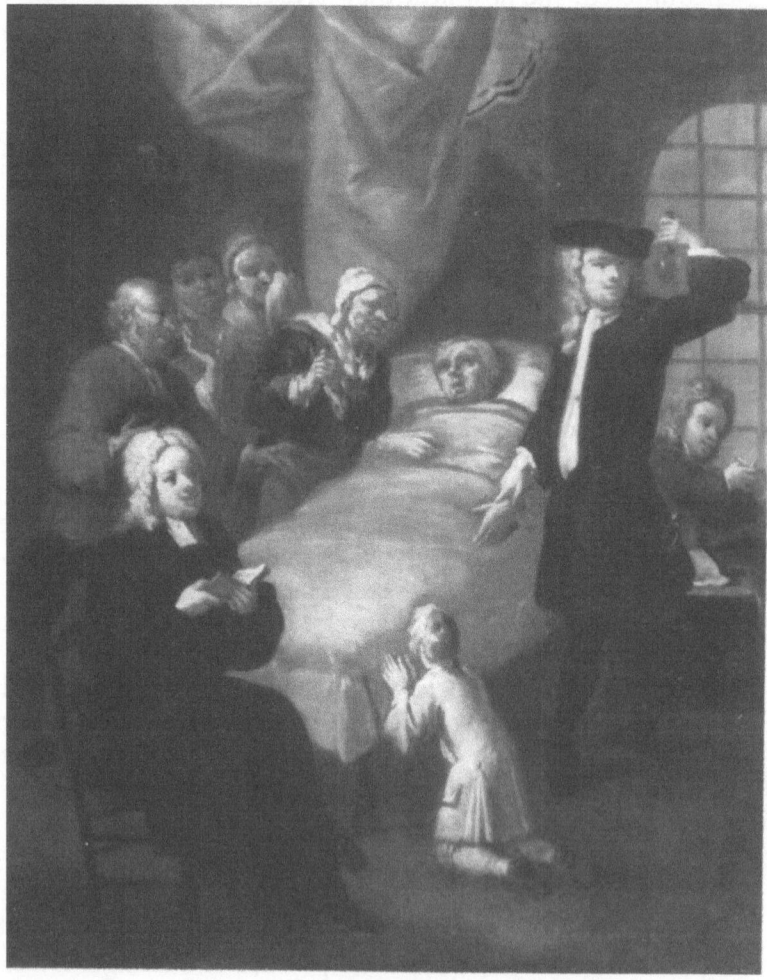

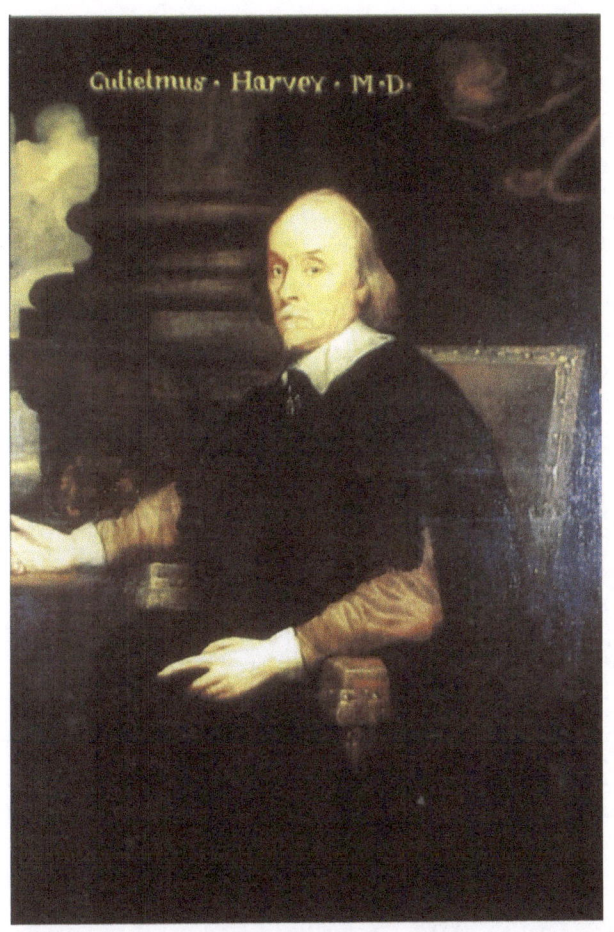

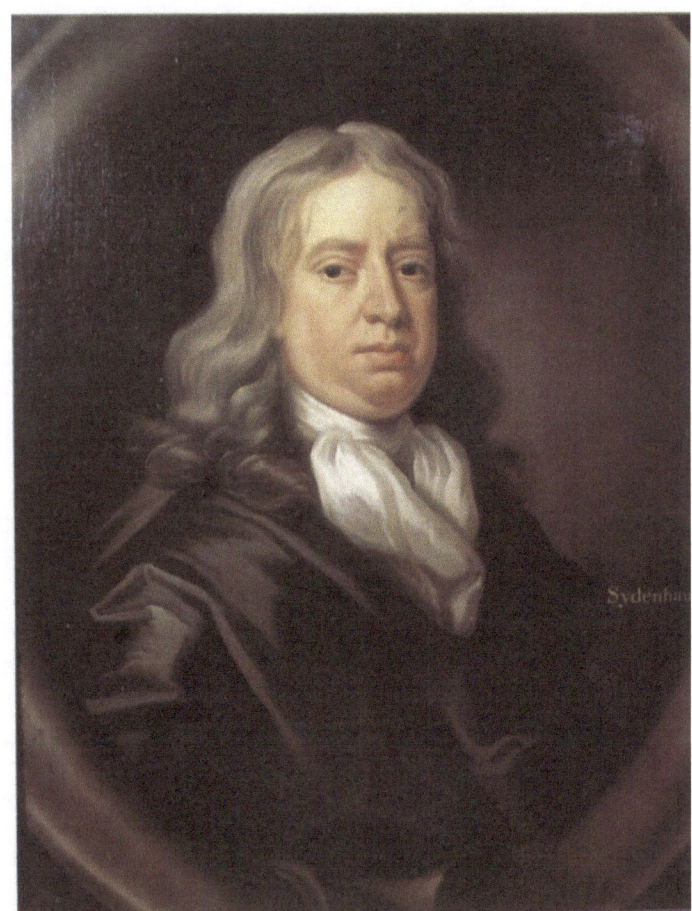

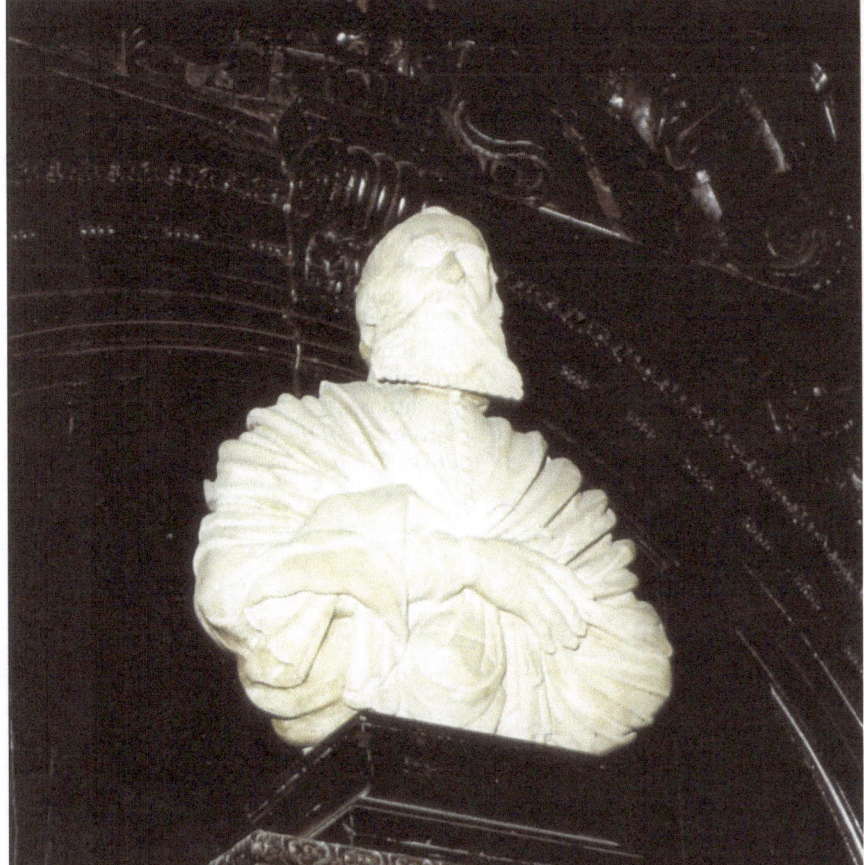

XXII
William Harvey (1578–1657),
circa 1650.
*By courtesy of the Treasurer,
Royal College of Physicians,
London.*

XXIII
Thomas Sydenham (1624–1689),
by Mary Beale.
*By courtesy of the Royal College
of Physicians, London.*

XXIV
The bust of Gideon de Laune, in
the Apothecaries' Hall.
*By courtesy of the Society of
Apothecaries.*

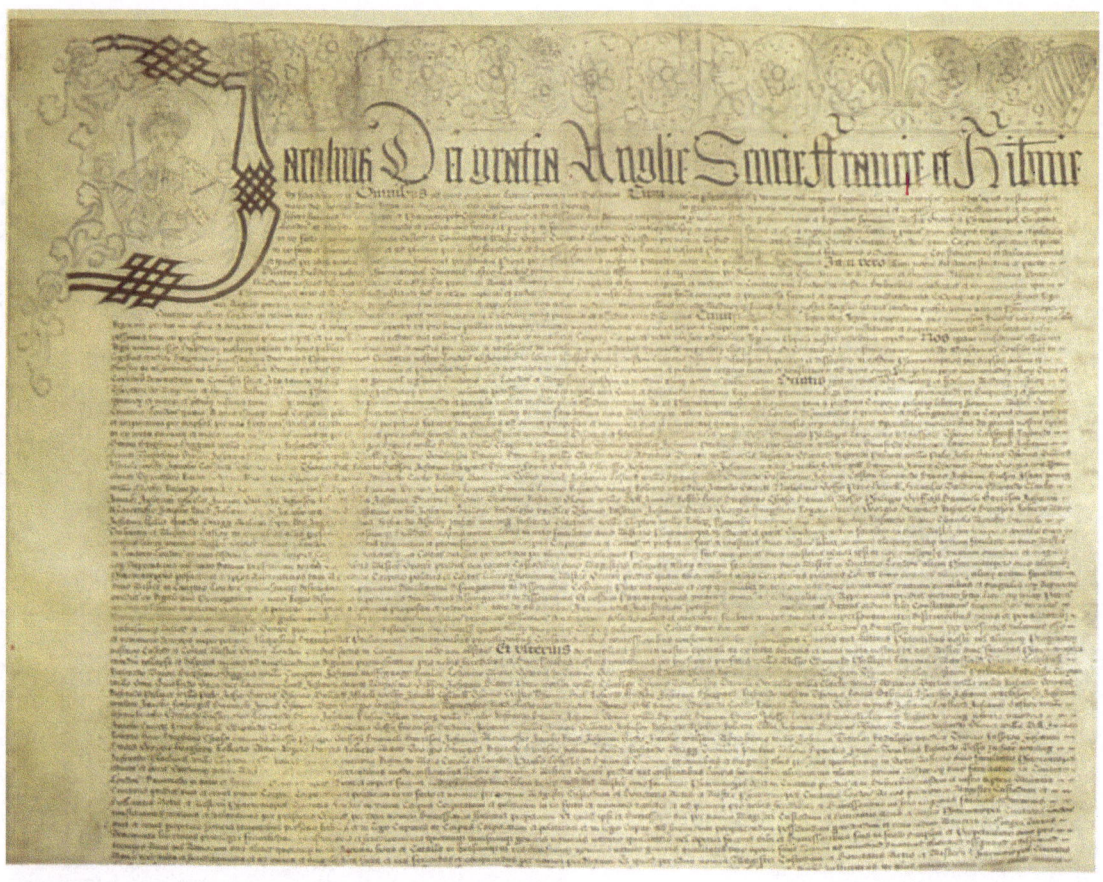

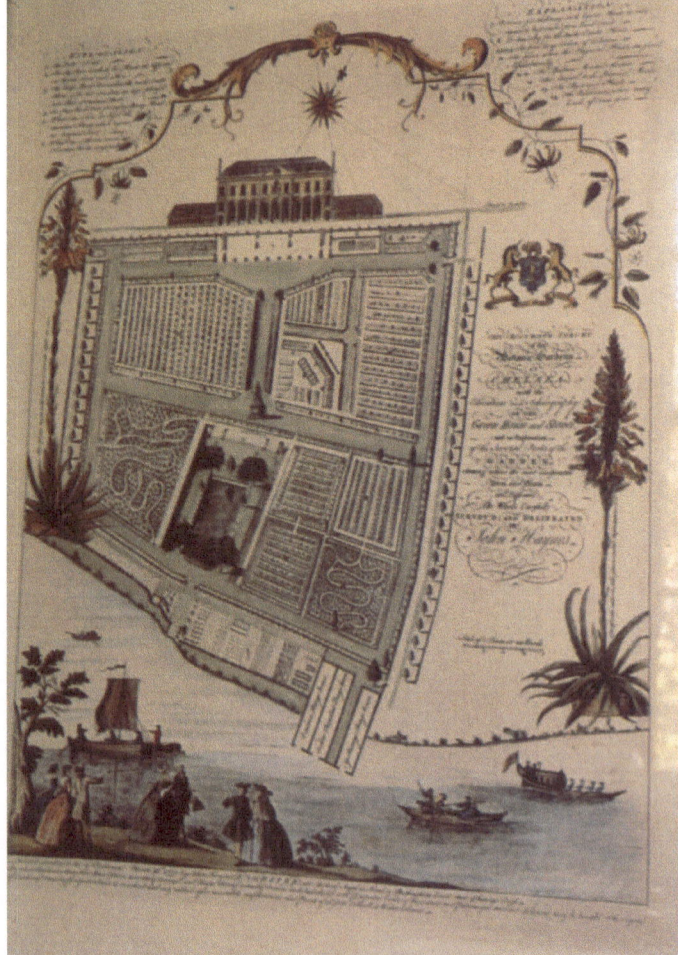

XXV
The Apothecaries' Charter
granted by James I in 1617.
*By courtesy of the Society of
Apothecaries.*

XXVI
The John Haynes map of the
Chelsea Physic Garden, 1753,
commissioned by the
Apothecaries from Haynes.
'An accurate survey of the
Botanic Gardens at Chelsea
and showing where the most
conspicuous trees and plants
are disposed'.
*By courtesy of the Chelsea
Physic Garden.*

The surgeons cared for some of the seriously ill in their own homes. It was therefore inadvisable that they should practise as barbers in case they infected their healthy customers. In the countryside the medical practitioners could not always visit the sick (figure 4) and some were nursed in the practitioners' own houses. The wife of John Hayne, an Exeter merchant, stayed for six weeks with Mr Forrester, a 'phisitian, neare Sherbourne'. His fee 'for lodging of the wife and maid, physic and his counsell' came to £4 10s, and she was so pleased with her treatment that she gave the doctor and his wife a 10s tip.

Advances in Diagnosis and Treatment

The scientific discoveries of the Stuart period gradually began to influence medical practice in the eighteenth century, particularly in the investigation of disease. John Floyer's minute watch for timing the pulse and respiration greatly improved the methods of diagnosis.

Floyer, however, in his book *The Physician's Pulse Watch* of 1707, lamented that Dr Harvey's work on the blood circulation which was expected to 'bring in great and general Innovations into the whole of Practice of Physik,' had had 'no such effect'. Indeed, Floyer's own clinical procedures were not accepted until their importance was stressed by the Dublin Physicians Robert Graves and William Stokes, over 100 years later.

Similarly, Auenbrugger's work on the value of percussion of the chest, contained in his book *Inventum Novum* of 1761, was totally forgotten until Corvisart rediscovered it in 1808.

Stephen Hales, the Rector of Teddington, measured the blood pressure of a horse, even though he was not medically trained. The doctors, however, made no attempt to apply this technique to their own clinical practice.

It was only after Morgagni, Corvisart and Laennec related signs and symptoms to pathological anatomical findings, that such discoveries could be utilised by the clinical practitioners in the diagnosis of disease.

Two major advances in treatment, however, received more prompt recognition. William Withering's (1741–1799) treatment of dropsy with digitalis, detailed in *An Account of the Foxglove and some of its medical Uses . . .*, became widely accepted. The doctors also appreciated the importance of Edward Jenner's (1749–1823) work on vaccinations (col. pl. XXVII).

The scientific thinking encouraged a completely new attitude to sanitation and hygiene. The Royal College of Physicians extended its interests to public health. Sir Hans Sloane, president of the College encouraged the introduction of the Gin Acts of 1736, 1751 and 1752 (figure 5). They were the forerunners of modern licensing laws, and aimed to curb drunkenness and so to reduce a great deal of distress and squalor and it also improved the quality of the gin! The College introduced a number of other public

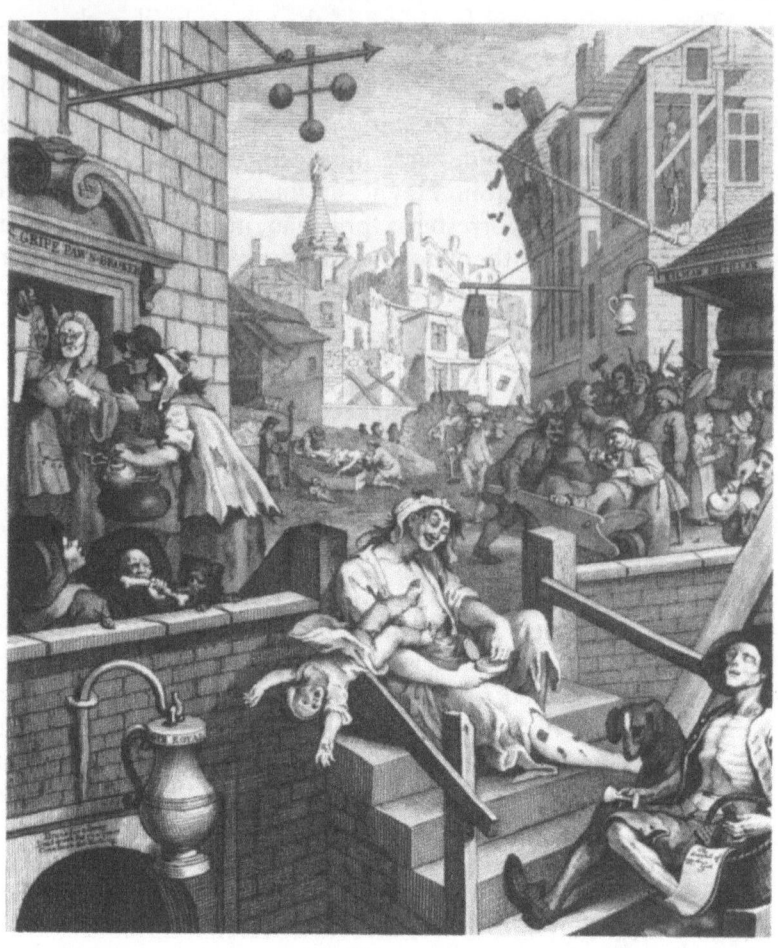

5. 'Gin Lane' or the Evils of
Drunkenness, by William Hogarth.
The whole sordid scene is shown: a
baby dropped by a drunken mother
surrounded by ruin caused by alcohol.
*By courtesy of the Bibliothèque
Nationale, Paris.*

health measures and played a major part in improving public
attitudes to health and hygiene.

John Hunter

John Hunter (1728–1793) (col. pl. XXVIII) combined his studies
in anatomy and physiology with practical surgery. He experi-
mented and observed disease and then tested the applicability of
his findings to practical surgery. Unfortunately, however, the
emphasis he placed on practical experiments led him once into
error. In an attempt to distinguish or unite the identities of
syphilis and gonorrhoea (a great contemporary argument) he
inoculated himself with what he believed to be gonorrhoeal pus
and developed a syphilitic primary chancre. From this experimental observation he drew what seemed to be the logical
conclusion.

As a teacher of surgery, John Hunter explained his craft in
terms of anatomy, physiology and pathology. It was this new

72

A

TREATISE

ON

THE BLOOD,

INFLAMMATION,

AND

GUN-SHOT WOUNDS,

BY THE LATE

JOHN HUNTER.

15 JUN 91

TO WHICH IS PREFIXED,

A SHORT ACCOUNT OF THE AUTHOR'S LIFE,

BY HIS BROTHER-IN-LAW,

EVERARD HOME.

LONDON:
Printed by John Richardson,
FOR GEORGE NICOL, BOOKSELLER TO HIS MAJESTY, PALL-MALL.
1794.

approach, combined with his active research into surgical pathology, shown in his *Treatise on the Blood, Inflammation and Gunshot Wounds* (1794) (figure 6), that improved the role of general surgery as part of general medical practice. This step helped unite the apothecary and surgeon, which marked the beginnings of the modern general practitioner in the next century.

6. The title page of John Hunter's *A Treatise on the Blood, Inflammation and Gunshot Wounds*, 1794.
By kind permission of the Royal College of Surgeons of England.

10
The
Apothecaries
Act of 1815

King George III, grandfather of Queen Victoria, was still reigning when the changes took place, defining apothecary and surgeon by examination and diploma, that gave good 'root of title' to the name 'physician and surgeon'. This was to appear on the brass plate of the Victorian general practitioner.

Medical Profession in the Early Nineteenth Century

THE SURGEONS

The Company of Surgeons was granted a royal charter in 1800 and changed its name to the Royal College of Surgeons. The by-laws of 1802 limited the diploma of the College to those over 22 years of age, but there was no longer any attempt to outline the geographical areas of the College's power or to establish a monopoly of control, as there had been earlier. The College officers were now more concerned with educating the surgeons and upgrading their position, but in practice only three courses of lectures were given between 1800 and 1813, one by Sir William Blizard, and two on comparative anatomy by Everard Home.

The Court of Examiners no longer insisted on an apprenticeship, accepting a four-year service in the shop of a chemist and druggist instead. The applicants were required only to have attended one course of lectures in anatomy and one in surgery, and until 1813 there was no need to have a hospital certificate of attendance in surgical practice.

THE APOTHECARIES

By the end of the eighteenth century there were apothecaries purely involved in dispensing; some dispensing and prescribing who thus practised medicine; and others practising surgery as well as medicine. The latter group often took the diploma of the new College of Surgeons which qualified them as surgeon-apothecaries. This group encroached on the traditional role of the physician, but it filled a social need by caring for the new middle class which the numerically few physicians were neither able nor willing to do. In 1814 Roberts Masters Kerrison stated that the surgeon-apothecaries had become 'the general practitioners throughout England and Wales: so that the health of at least 19 out of every 20 patients is now regulated by them alone'.

Dr James Parkinson (1755–1824) came of a family of surgeon-apothecaries in rural Shoreditch. His father, John, was a shopkeeper as well as anatomical warden of the Surgeons' Company. James attended John Hunter's lectures, transcribed them in shorthand and they were later published by James's son John. He wrote many books besides his famous 'Essay on the Shaking Palsy'. *Medical Admonitions* is an interesting collection of his practical views. He discusses ophthalmia neonatorum as a cause of blindness and recommends early surgery for breast cancer. *The*

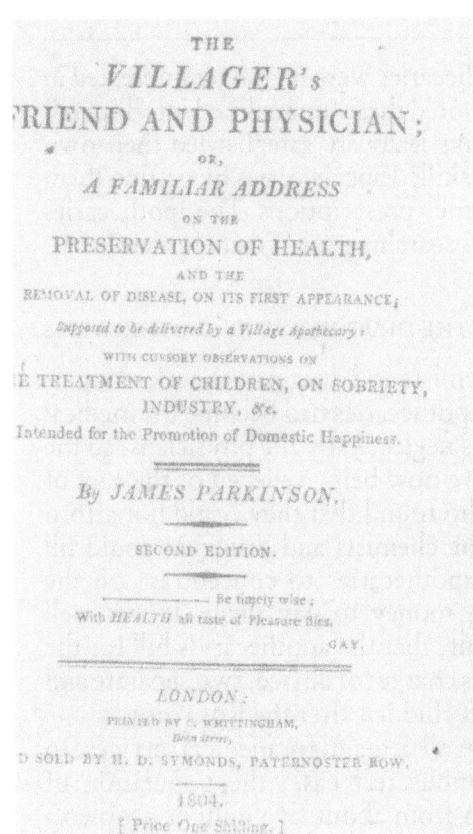

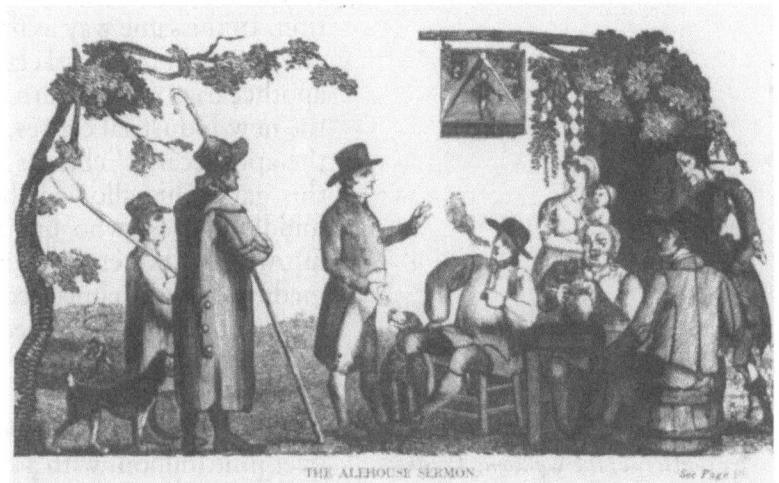

Villager's Friend and Physician (figures 1, 2 and 3) is a simplified version of *Medical Admonitions* and is one of the 'Home Doctor' type of book which became very popular in the nineteenth century.

CHEMISTS AND DRUGGISTS

As the apothecaries became increasingly involved in the practice of medicine, the new 'chemists and druggists' at the bottom of the medical hierarchy, filled the gap left by the apothecaries who were less concerned with the preparation and sale of drugs.

The chemists and druggists had their origins in the grocery business, but had concentrated on the new trade in chemicals and drugs that had arisen in the seventeenth century. At this stage few of them actually made the drugs they sold, they simply supplied them to the apothecaries (figure 4 and col. pl. XXIX). They became known as drugmen or 'drugsters' and later as 'chemists and druggists'.

These specialists in drugs and chemicals increased in number to meet the retail market's demand for supplies in which the apothecaries had lost interest. There was also an overall need for more retailers, and as a result the chemists and druggists became as numerous as the surgeon-apothecaries in some towns. This pattern was not repeated on the continent, however, where the apothecaries have retained their role as retailers.

1. The title page of James Parkinson's *The Villager's Friend and Physician*, second edition 1804.
   By courtesy of the Wellcome Trustees.

2. 'The Alehouse Sermon', frontispiece from James Parkinson's *The Villager's Friend and Physician*.
   By courtesy of the Wellcome Trustees.

Although most of the apothecaries were no longer interested in supplying medicines they resented these 'unqualified interlopers', particularly as they had always jealously safeguarded their own standards. They irritated the skilled apothecaries by getting them up at night to translate emergency prescriptions. The apothecaries also joked about the druggists searching for 'Tinct ejusdem'.

THE RELATIONSHIP BETWEEN THE DRUGGISTS AND APOTHECARIES

It was now the turn of the chemists and druggists to seek recognition. In the same way as the apothecaries had become the medical attendants of the social classes neglected by the physicians, so the apothecaries in their turn were now being relieved of the care of the new industrial classes, who found that they could not afford the apothecaries' charges. The chemists and druggists could fill this gap. This allowed the apothecaries to concentrate on the middle classes, who had the money to pay them. It was well known, but not entirely unfair, that the apothecary's bill for the medicine always concealed his charge for advice, two separate and distinct charges having been forbidden after the Rose case.

There was also a greater overall demand for medical services. In the 100 years since that famous test case, the population of England and Wales had risen from about five million people to over nine million, with a shift of workers to the industrial north.

3. Pages from James Parkinson's book.
By courtesy of the Wellcome Trustees.

6

and scandalous imputations of ignorance, or neglect.

Nor is this all; recollect with how little consideration for his comfort, is the time, as well as the labour, of a village apothecary trifled with. Have you to consult your lawyer, or to employ any other man almost in the village, you will require his attendance, at that time which may best suit his convenience; but should a trifling rash on the skin, which has hardly excited your attention for a week or two, at last induce you to call for the attendance of your apothecary, the application will frequently be deferred to the close of the day: nor will the roughest and most tempestuous weather excuse his attendance, which will, in general, be thought necessary to be insisted on *directly*, to give energy and effect to your message; not considering that he who calls wolf unnecessarily, may call in vain, when in real danger.—Excuse these remarks, which may not, at first sight, appear calculated so much for your benefit, as for that of the apothecary; but you should consider that, in proportion as you manifest a regard for his comfort, you will, of course, render him zealous and interested for your welfare. In general, in proportion as you attend to his convenience, will he be enabled to apply himself to procure you benefit. Thus, when your message is not sent before

7

he sets off for his usual rounds, you not only give him the trouble of pacing over a mile or two of ground, which he has already trodden; but your summons taking him out of his regular course, perhaps in the midst of the hurry of business, it is far from improbable, that your concerns, from the crowd of various circumstances then engaging his thoughts, cannot obtain that attention, which he may be anxious to give them.

Delaun Reviv'd,

Viz.

A Plain and short discourse of that *Famous*

DOCTOR'S PILLS,

Their Use and Virtues.

VVith Choice Receipts for the Cure of the *Scurvy, Dropsy, Jaundies, Venereal* and other Diseases.

Before I speak to this Famous Medicine, I will declare who Delaun was; Then, the Price of his Pill and how to take it, and of its several Virtues in order, in such Plain words, as the weakest capacity may understand:

And I intreat those who hope for help hereby, would throughly *Read* this short book, and observe my Directions for their own good and the Authors's Credit.

This *Famous* Author was not like any the *Quacks* of this Age, whom the Honourable *London Colleagues* could comptrol, as they did *Bromfield of Fetter Lane* most deservedly, and compell'd him to pay *Forty marks*; for that, *who Delaun was* that he, though the chief of the *Pill-sellers*, was never bred to Physick, or had Learning enough to understand his *Accidence*; Mr. *Scott* in *Grubstreet* Attorney for the Colledge, who prosecuted many others, will averr this truth: which, if *Bromfield* (or any

(11)

qualified only to compound, not daring, (in seven years more) to administer or prescribe *a dose of Physick*: I leave it to any sober man to judge, but, since [...] I will desist.

In Laudem Authoris.

Med'cine Apollo *clayms, Spagyrick Art*
Is Thine Great Laun; Now Chymists do not Thwart
The Galenists; all Reconcil'd by this
Thy Posthume Pill, the Rich and Poor Mans bliss.
Sr. *Robert Sprignel* Knight and Baronet, one of *Delaun's* Grandsons

*So shone the Sun, and Python did destroy,
As you those Ills which Mankind do annoy,
Do Conquer, since these Arts you do Employ.*
A. Oldis Delaun's God-son.

These Pills are Sold

At *Delaun's Head* a Feather-maker in *Black-Fryers*, next door to my former Habitation by *Ludgate.* By Mr. *Horn* at the *North Entrance* of the *Old Exchange.* Mrs. *Hope* at the *South Entrance.* Mr. *Leech* at the *Crown* in *Cornhill.* Mr. [...] under St. *Dunstans* Church. Mr. *Carter* at the *flying Horse* in *Fleetstreet*, Mr. *Battersby* at *Thavies Inn* Gate, all Booksellers. Mr. *Leeson* in *Bow lane* the Famous Tooth-drawer. Mr. *Searle* in *Fye-places Corner* the Great Operator in *Deafness.* Mr. *Appleby* at the *Apple Tree* in *for Sale Piccadilly*, near the *French Church.* Mr. *Charles Branden* Cheesemonger in *Clare Market.* The *five Bells* in *Chancery Lane*, Cutler. Mr. *Montague* in *Fleetstreet*, Tobacconist. Mr. *Morgan* the Kings Grocer in *Henrietta street Covent Garden.* Mr. *Weatherspoon* Barber Chyrurgion in *Long Acre.* Mr. *Eads* Distiller in *Leather lane.* Capt. *Grant* in Moor-fields. Mr. *Lovell* on *London bridge*, (Distillers.) *Dawes* Coffee-house at *Smithfield Bars.* Mr. *Hatton* Vintner. Mr. *Seager* Tobacconist. Mr. *Parruck* Grocer. Mrs. *Harvey* Thred-shop, (these four in *Holbourn.*) Mr. *Fages* in St. *James's* Market, Grocer. Mrs. *Milward* at *Westminster Hall* Gate. Mrs. *Rookes* in *Kingstreet*, and at her shop at *White Hall* Milliner. Mr. *Only* Grocer in *Red-Cross street.* Mr. *Hubbert* Tinman in *Upper Shadwell.* Mr. *Smith* over against the *Kings Bench* at the *Bird Cage* in *Southwark.* Mr. *Smith*

Attempts to Reform the Medical Profession

THE GENERAL PHARMACEUTICAL ASSOCIATION

In June 1794, at the *Crown and Anchor* in the Strand, an effort was made to safeguard the status of the apothecary, to regulate his practice, 'and to restrain ignorant and unqualified persons from practising at all'. Practically minded apothecaries were more concerned about their loss of income. They had already impressively calculated that if the profits made by the sneaky infringements of the druggists were to be divided among the apothecaries where it rightfully belonged, 'everyone would have an addition of nearly £200 a year to his present income'. They also complained, 'taxes have been doubled, house-rent has been doubled, the price of almost every material has been doubled, but the price of medicines . . . has had scarcely any advance in any place'.

In an attempt to safeguard their interests, the apothecaries formed the General Pharmaceutical Association of Great Britain, with an annual subscription of one guinea. The Association collected evidence showing the incompetence of the chemists and druggists, and then approached the College of Physicians, the Society of Apothecaries and the Corporation of Surgeons. The Worshipful Society of Apothecaries, however, was so implacably opposed to its proposals, that the Association was effectively destroyed.

4. An eighteenth century advertisement for De Laune's pills.
By courtesy of the Wellcome Trustees.

77

THE COLLEGE'S PROPOSALS

The need for an ordering, for a definition of the skills of the component members of 'the body of physick', was recognised. In a more comprehensive way than the particular interests of the General Pharmaceutical Association, Dr Edward Harrison, MD (Edinburgh) was concerned with the whole structure of the profession. He spoke up at a meeting of the Lincolnshire Benevolent Medical Society, when his proposals were enthusiastically received. They were far more acceptable to the majority of practitioners than were those of the Royal College of Physicians, which had been proposed by Dr John Latham in 1804, embellished by the College and published in 1806.

This plan put forward that the country should be divided into 16 districts each under the control of a resident physician. His salary of £500 was to be found from a levy of 2 guineas per annum from each qualified practitioner. His function was to examine candidates who did not have any recognised qualifications, and with the help of assessors, he had to decide whether or not they were fit to practise. The College prepared a Bill which set out its age requirements and the type of training and qualifications needed for all physicians, surgeons, apothecaries, chemists and druggists, in England and Wales. Through this bill, the College (figure 5) hoped finally to achieve its ambition of controlling the whole of medical practice.

5. The Royal College of Physicians, Warwick Lane, 1804.
By courtesy of the Royal College of Physicians, London

6. 'The Rapacious Quack'. Anonymous English mezzotint published by Carrington Bowles, London, in the eighteenth century. In the Wellcome Institute.
By courtesy of the Wellcome Trustees.

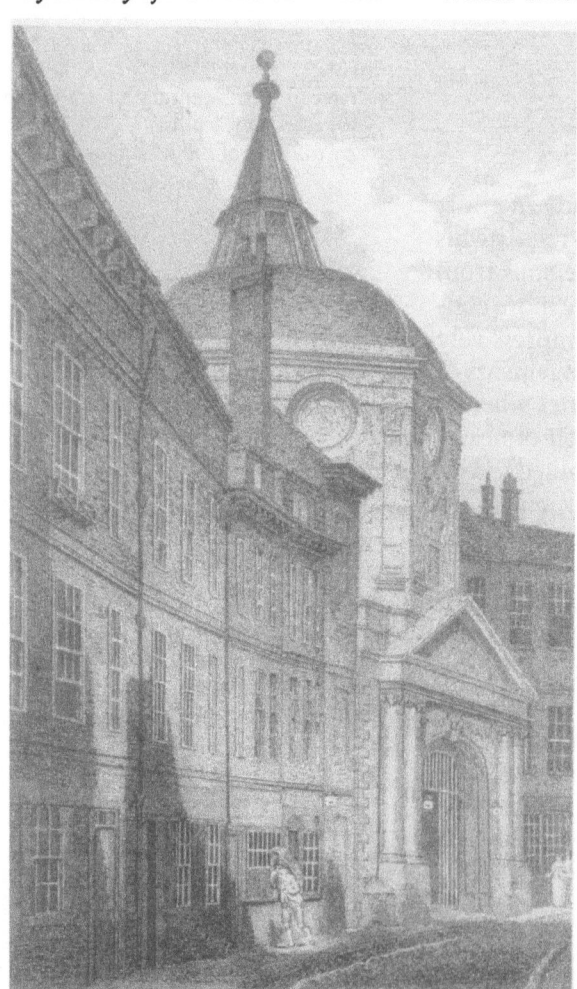

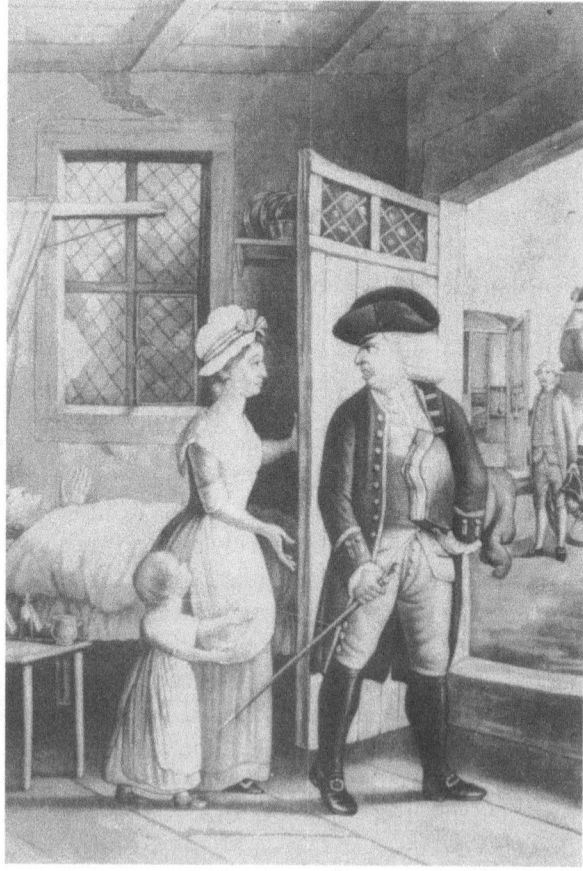

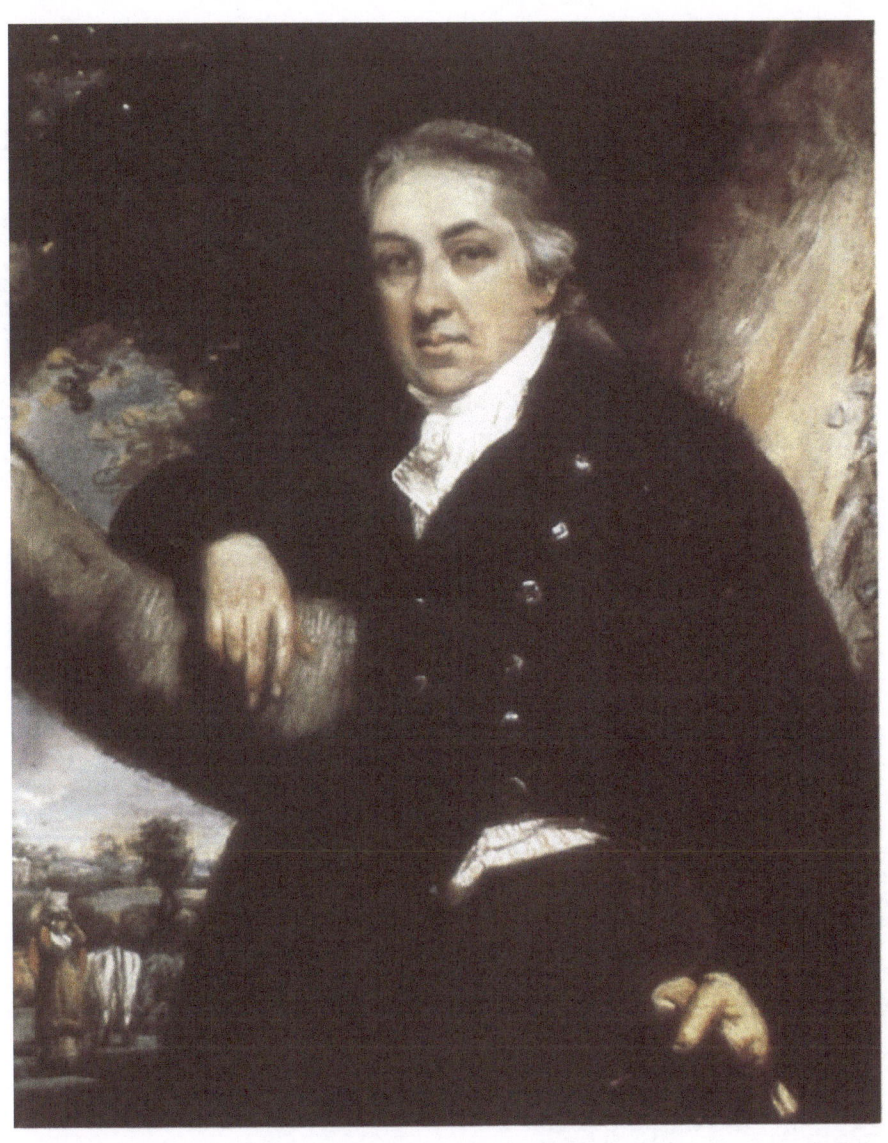

XXVII
Portrait of Edward Jenner, 1800, by J. R. Smith, with a view of Berkeley in the background.
By courtesy of the Wellcome Trustees.

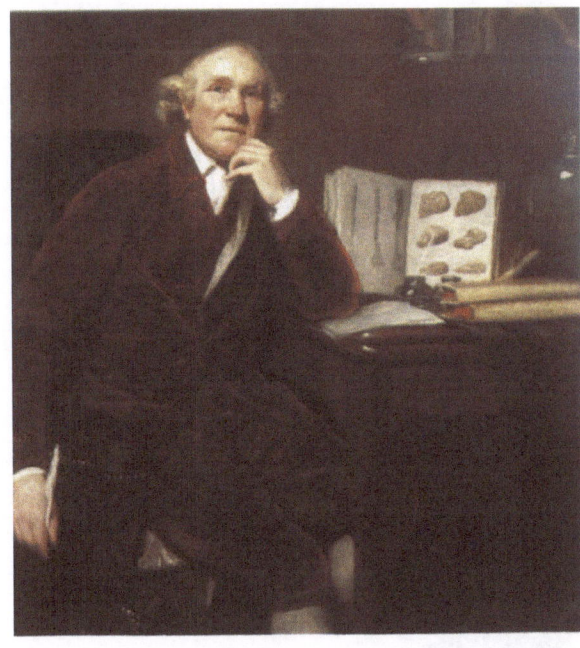

XXVIII
Portrait of John Hunter (1728–1793), by J. Reynolds, 1786.
By kind permission of the Royal College of Surgeons of England.

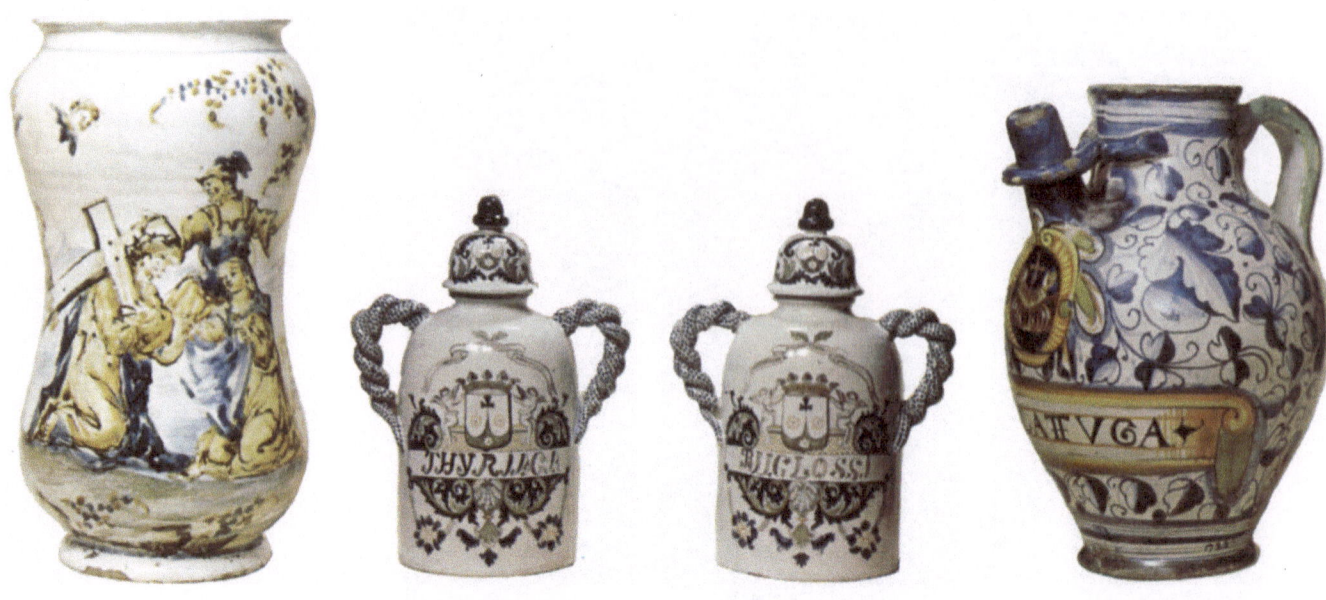

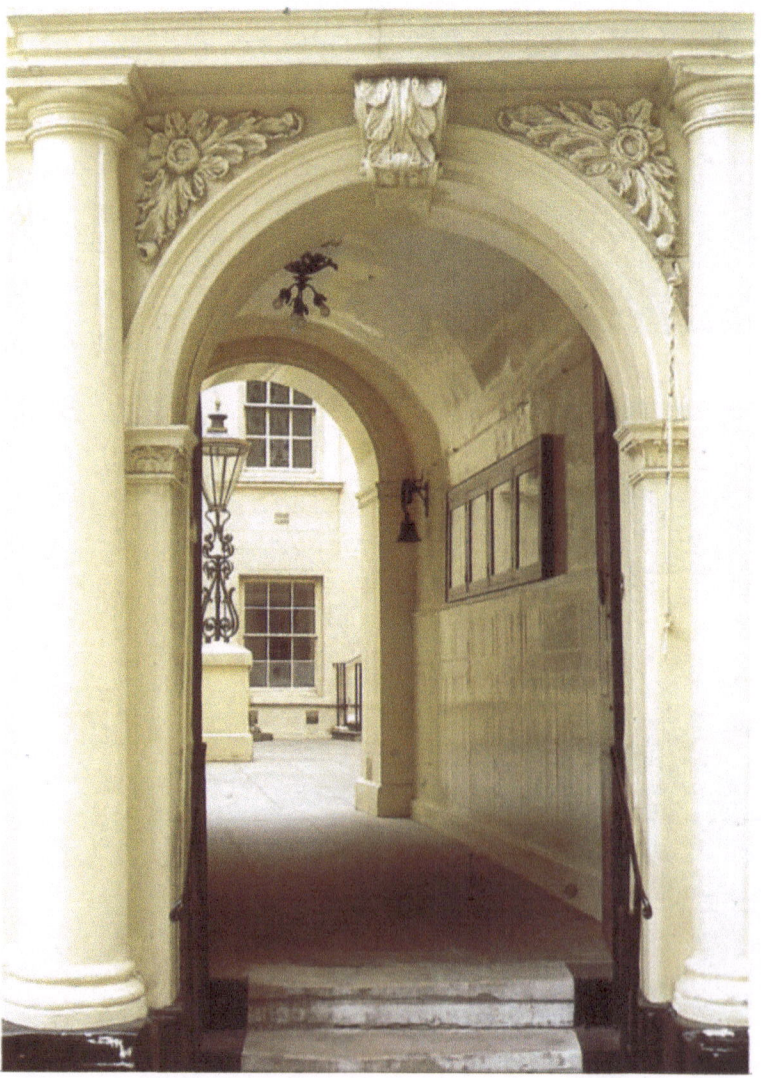

XXIX
Drug jars. 1. Albarello, one of a set of six Istoriato paintings of biblical scenes inscribed with the beacon mark of Genoa. 2. Pair of large drug jars (French, probably eighteenth century). 3. Syrup-shape drug jar (Italian, probably Tuscan sixteenth century).
By courtesy of the Wellcome Trustees.

XXX
The entrance to the courtyard of the Apothecaries' Hall, London. The present buildings date from the seventeenth century after the Great Fire of London.
Photograph by the author.

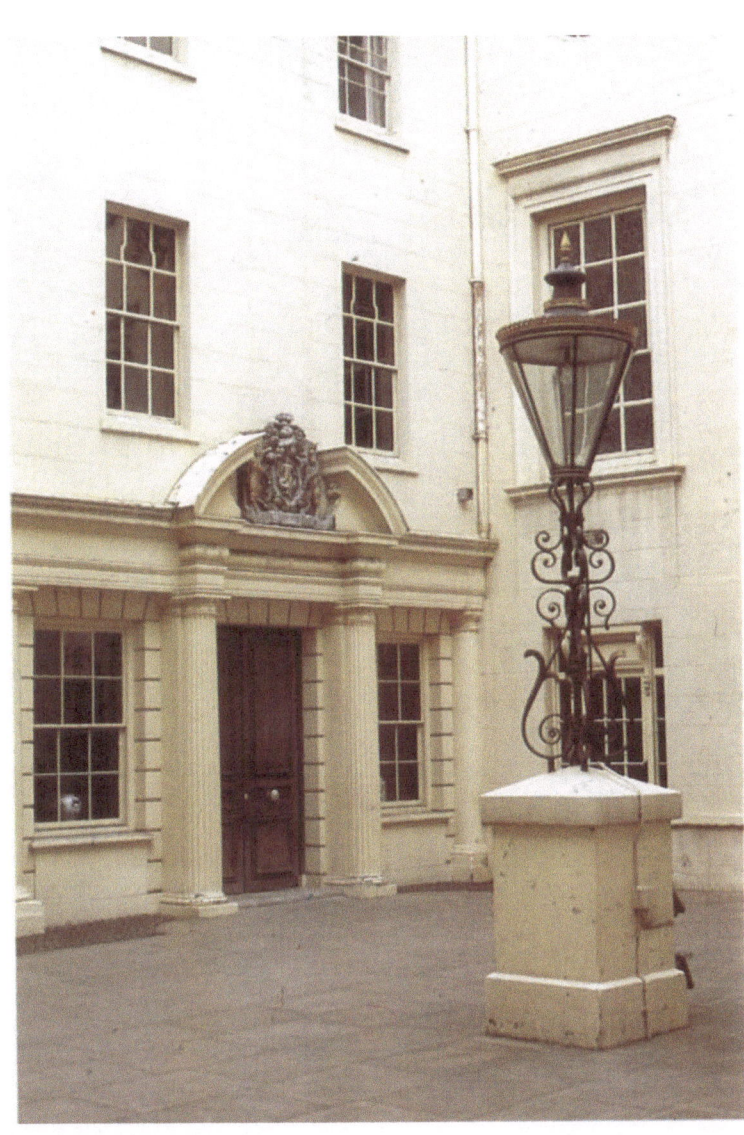

XXXI
The courtyard to the
Apothecaries' Hall, London.
The Arms show Apollo the
god of medicine bestride a
serpent. The supporters are
unicorns and the crest a
rhinoceros. The horn of the
unicorn had a reputation as an
antidote for poison. The horn
of the rhinoceros was a cheaper
substitute.
Photograph by the author.

XXXII
The Royal College of Surgeons
of England.
*By kind permission of the
Royal College of Surgeons of
England.*

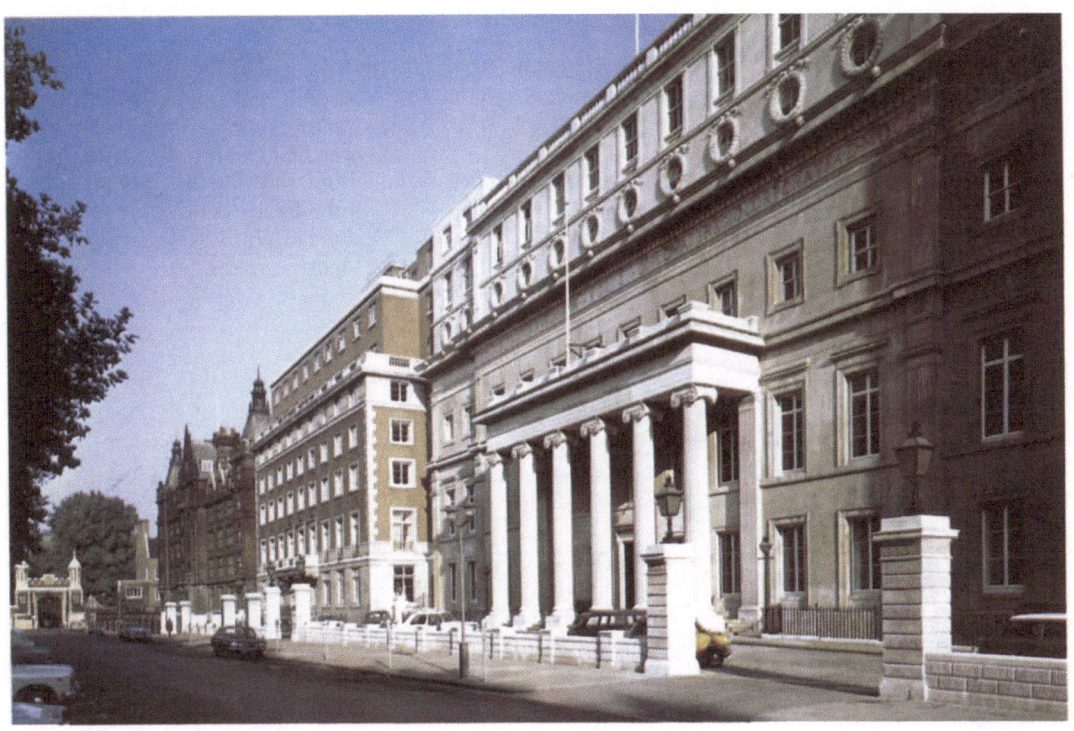

July 25th 1816. –

189 MR. *John Keats of full age* — CANDIDATE for a CERTIFICATE to practise as an APOTHECARY in *the country*. —

An APPRENTICE to MR. *Thomas Hammond of Edmonton* APOTHECARY for *5* Years.

TESTIMONIAL from *Mr Thos Hammond* . —

LECTURES.

2 COURSES on ANATOMY and PHYSIOLOGY.
2 ——— THEORY and PRACTICE of MEDICINE.
2 ——— CHEMISTRY.
1 ——— MATERIA MEDICA.

HOSPITAL ATTENDANCE.

6 MONTHS at *Guy's & St Thomas's* . —

as

MONTHS at

168 *examined by Mr Brande & approved*

John Keats. Poet

XXXIII
The first Court of Examiners'
Book showing the entry for
John Keats, 1816.
*By courtesy of the Society of
Apothecaries.*

THE ASSOCIATED FACULTY

Dr Harrison blandly stated that his plan aimed to reserve the practice of medicine to 'youths of reputable birth, and liberal education', and 'to prevent the admission of mean and low persons' to the profession (figure 6). Despite this, it was a comprehensive plan which won free postage from the Treasury and the sympathy of William Pitt and Spencer Percival. He was also given encouragement by a number of eminent people in the medical profession: Sir Joseph Banks (1743–1820) the President of the Royal Society, J.C.Forster the Master of the Royal College of Surgeons, and surprisingly Sir George Baker (1722–1809) the President of the Royal College of Physicians.

His supporters formed a group called the 'Associated Faculty', which met at Sir Joseph Banks' house, and drew up a Bill 'for better regulating the Practice of Physic'. The main points were:

1. Physicians should be at least 24 years of age, be graduates of a university in the UK, and have studied physic for five years.

2. Surgeons should be at least 23 years of age and be licensed by one of the corporations of surgeons after serving a five-year apprenticeship and studying anatomy and surgery for two years in a medical school.

3. Apothecaries should be at least 21 and have studied physic in a school for one year after serving a five-year apprenticeship.

4. No man should practise midwifery unless he had attended anatomical lectures and received instruction from an experienced accoucheur for one year.

5. Female midwives should obtain a certificate of proficiency from an obstetrician.

6. Chemists and druggists should serve a five-year apprenticeship.

7. Every person entering upon the practice of any branch of the profession should pay a fine on admission to the register of qualified practitioners.

8. There should be no interference with those already practising.

There was to be a medical register (with an annual fee) for all duly qualified physicians, surgeons, midwives, apothecaries, veterinary practitioners, chemists and druggists, and vendors of medicines. Commissioners were to be appointed to enforce the Act and they were also to be given authority to set up hospitals, medical schools and libraries.

Harrison's Bill was eventually defeated by the College who feared that it would displace the traditional supremacy of the physicians:

The real design and tendency of Dr Harrison's proposals are less directed to the amelioration of medical practice than to the subversion of the existing authorities in Physic, and the depression of the rights, the rank, and the importance of the Physician.

79

The Society of Apothecaries was not willing to give any encouragement; it prudently declined to given an opinion on what reforms were necessary in other parts of the profession, but felt quite competent to control its own members.

Harrison abandoned his Bill in 1811, having received this advice from an Edinburgh physician:

Before your proposed reform can be accomplished, physic must be made more perfect, physicians more honest, statesmen more enlightened, and the bulk of mankind much wiser and better than they are at present, or have ever been, or are likely to become in our time.

The main reason for his failure lay in the entrenched attitudes of the three great governing bodies—the College of Physicians, the College of Surgeons, and the Society of Apothecaries—despite the enlightened support shown by their leaders.

THE ASSOCIATION OF APOTHECARIES AND SURGEON-APOTHECARIES

In 1812, the Government decided to impose a heavy tax on glass. This obviously threatened the apothecaries' incomes, as most of their medicines were sold in bottles. It was a threat which rallied the apothecaries together and somehow another Edinburgh graduate, Dr Anthony Todd Thomson, succeeded once more in introducing the subject of medical reform.

The Association of Apothecaries and Surgeon-Apothecaries was formed to protect the status and income of the apothecaries against the encroachment of the chemists and druggists. The reformers limited themselves to the control of apothecaries, surgeon-apothecaries, midwives and compounders of medicine, leaving the physicians and surgeons to manage their own affairs. At first, their well-meaning efforts met with sullen indifference from the Colleges and Society of Apothecaries, but this eventually turned to opposition when they attempted to put forward a Bill. They were also attacked by the now powerful 'Chemists and Druggists of the Metropolis' under the guidance of William Allen of Plough Court (figure 7), John Savory of Bond Street, John Bell of Oxford Street and W. B. Hudson of the Haymarket. These chemists were later to become household names. The chemists and druggists succeeded in preventing any outside control of their interests.

The Association did not give up and under the chairmanship of George Mann Burrows it eventually succeeded in placating the opposition to place the control of the apothecaries in the hands of the Society of Apothecaries.

THE APOTHECARIES ACT OF 1815

The Apothecaries Act of 1815 enlarged the Charter of the Society of Apothecaries in London and announced it was 'for better regulating the Practice of Apothecaries throughout England and

Wales'. Those persons not already in practice on 1 August, 1815, but who desired to do so 'must submit themselves for examination'. They had to be 21 years of age, 'have served a five-year apprenticeship, and produce testimonials of a sufficient medical education and of good moral character'. Assistants likewise had to be examined and certified. An annual register was to be kept and penalties for failure to compound medicines prescribed by a licensed physician included being 'struck off' for the third offence. Fines for unregistered practice were laid down. Clauses 28 and 29 made it clear that the Act should not affect chemists and druggists in:

the buying, preparing, compounding, dispensing, and vending drugs, medicines, and medicinable compounds, wholesale or retail . . . privileges of the universities of Oxford and Cambridge, and the Royal College of Physicians and Surgeons shall not be affected by this Act.

Contemporary reaction was less than enthusiastic by those who had hoped for a sweeping reform of medical practice. The apothecaries were still clearly subordinate to the physicians, even to the extent of being compelled to dispense their prescriptions. The mark of the tradesman was there for all to see in the apprenticeship requirement.

Nevertheless, the Act was of great importance in shaping the future of general medical practice. The qualification of the good general practitioner had become MRCS, LSA and the hitherto conservative Court of the Society of Apothecaries was to take a leading part, supported by the Royal College of Surgeons, in establishing the standard of practice.

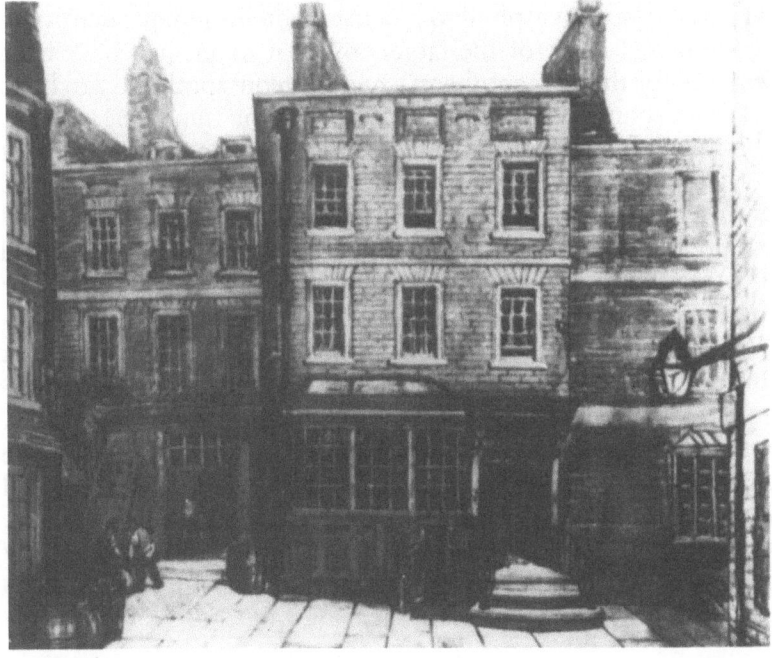

7. The pharmacy of Allen & Hanburys at No. 2 Plough Court, Lombard Street, in 1715.
By courtesy of Allen & Hanburys Ltd.

11
Nineteenth Century Educational Reform of General Practice

The Apothecaries Act

DEFINITION OF APOTHECARIAL PRACTICE

The Act showed all the signs of a hasty construction and had in fact been passed by only one vote on the last day of a session in a depleted House.

The nearest the Act of 1815 came to explaining the practice of the new apothecary was the clause making him in effect 'only to be the phisician's cooke'. The fifth clause, inserted expressly at the demand of the College of Physicians, made it:

the duty of every person using or exercising the art and mystery of an apothecary to prepare with exactness and to dispense such medicines as may be directed for the sick by any physician lawfully licensed.

In defining one of his duties, this clearly indicated his menial status. Unfortunately, it did not define apothecarial practice. It therefore followed that the above requirement could only apply to those foolish enough to call themselves apothecaries.

It would appear that anyone who was not an apothecary could perform many of the functions of a general medical practitioner without contravening the law. These points were not missed in the medical press. The *Lancet* in 1826 commented that 'attending and prescribing for the sick are not once alluded to as forming parts of an Apothecary's duties'. It might therefore be better simply not to call oneself an apothecary, if by so doing the main result was to expose oneself to the penal clauses of the Act.

The Society of Apothecaries (col. pls. XXX and XXXI) was felt to be a society of tradesmen, only one stage removed from the grocers. By obtaining its licence, the practitioner subordinated himself to the College of Physicians. Its longest tradition was in the selling and compounding of drugs, although its members had for some time past aspired to practise medicine independently. In London and some of the larger towns it might just have been possible for the new apothecary and surgeon-apothecary to hope to practise medicine without at the same time engaging in pharmacy. In the crowded cities there were many among the rest of their colleagues who were happy to continue the sale of drugs. In the country at large, anyone engaged in the healing art would usually be forced by circumstance to dispense for himself, as well as prescribe, whether he called himself physician, surgeon or apothecary. The Act did not define medical practice.

The Act had eventually to be tested by the judges, and not surprisingly they decided that legally qualified general practitioners required the licentiateship of the Society of Apothecaries. In another judgement of 1834, an apothecary was defined as 'one who professes to judge of internal diseases by its symptoms and applies himself to cure disease by medicine'. The day of the apothecary in general medical practice had arrived. It had already been ruled that an apothecary could recover fees for attendance as well as medicines in 1830.

ASSOCIATION WITH TRADE

The compulsory association with trade through the Society of Apothecaries was resented by many. They felt that it was the universities, and not a city gild, that should have been given the power to regulate the qualifications of medical practitioners as was the custom in Europe.

There is no doubt that the necessity for an indenture was disliked. The apprentice was bound for five years in the sum of £35 not to:

haunt taverns, inns or alehouses . . . At cards, dice, tables or any other unlawful games he shall not play, nor from the service of his said master day or night shall absent himself, but in all things as an honest and faithful apprentice shall and will demean and behave himself toward his said master.

If he carried out his time and duty faithfully he could apply for £20 toward the setting up or the carrying on of his own business. Trade was very much in mind in the years before and after the Act.

The five-year apprenticeship clause was a mixed blessing. It was argued that the practical instruction it gave could be gained in a fraction of the time and that it interfered in the obtaining of a general liberal education by the apprentices. The most that the Society was able to do to accommodate this criticism was to allow

1. St Bartholomew's Hospital, circa 1829. *Mary Evans Picture Library.*

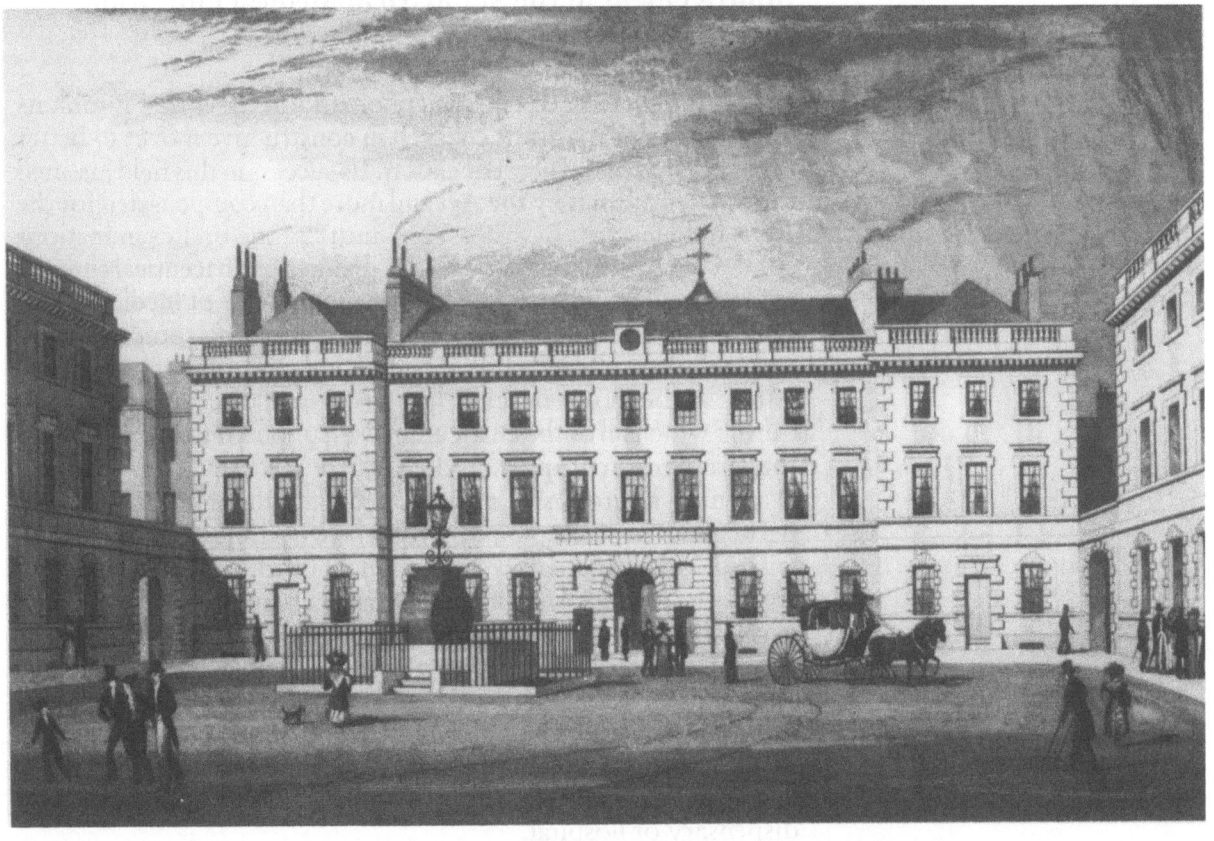

the hospital training to count as part of the five-year apprenticeship. Before the beginning of Queen Victoria's reign some 100 hospitals and 40 schools had been inspected by the Society of Apothecaries and approved for teaching.

The College of Surgeons (col. pl. XXXII) had already tried to rid itself of the stigma of any association with trade, by severing its traditional links with the City and pointedly ignoring apprenticeship requirements. Many surgeons, who had both qualifications, preferred not to disclose their LSA. Medical graduates of the Scottish universities found themselves precluded from general dispensing practice in England and Wales, unless they were prepared to undergo the five year apprenticeship required of an apothecary who wished to take the LSA; only this would give him the right to practise. The Society of Apothecaries forgot its earlier declarations of humility not to extend its powers to other branches of the profession. It threatened to implement the Act against the graduates of the Scottish universities. Many students had gone to Scotland, attracted by the quality of the course in medicine, surgery and midwifery. Surgeons, too, had to be careful not to overstep the mark, for a surgeon however well qualified in surgery who was not in addition licensed by the Society, was not permitted to administer medicine for non-surgical conditions.

Improvement in the Standard of Medical Education

THE SOCIETY OF APOTHECARIES

It was to the credit of the Society of Apothecaries that it took its new role seriously, for it engaged in constructive moves to better the standards of medical education. Its success in this field justified the powers given it by the Act and more than compensated for the Act's deficiencies. Between 1815 and 1840 the oral examinations conducted by the Society, covering Latin, pharmaceutical chemistry and materia medica, the theory and practice of medicine (but not surgery or midwifery), were recognised as comprehensive and fair. A candidate's final examination consisted of a viva voce lasting at the most one and a half to one and three quarter hours, during which all of the curriculum was supposed to be covered by the examiners (col. pl. XXXIII). These were twelve in number, examining in groups of three. One of the three questioned any particular candidate, but the other two could join in if they wished. If the candidate was not thought up to standard, examiners from other groups were invited to take part and no-one was failed except by a majority of all the examiners. This final test came at the end of approved courses, attested by certificates of attendance at the hospitals or dispensaries and at the lectures. There were to be three lectures and demonstrations on anatomy and physiology, three on the theory and practice of medicine, three on chemistry, and three on materia medica with six months' attendance at a dispensary or hospital.

THE COLLEGE OF SURGEONS

After the 1815 Act the College of Surgeons gradually brought their requirements into line with those of the Society of Apothecaries. Their standards of hospital teaching were, if anything, higher than those required by the Society of Apothecaries. Certificates of attendance upon the surgical practice of a hospital, and of lectures on anatomy, physiology, theory and practice of surgery and the performance of dissections were required. In 1828 the College added two courses of lectures on the obstetric art and science. The final examination was in anatomy and surgery. The attempts to tighten these standards by insisting that only those anatomy lectures given in the winter session would be recognised by the College, caused a furore because it ruined attendance at the excellent private summer courses. In 1824 the Court of Examiners decided to recognise only the schools of surgery at London, Dublin, Edinburgh, Glasgow and Aberdeen. This cut out the newest provincial schools and led to such a spirited indignation by Thomas Wakely, editor of the *Lancet*, that it resulted in their eventual recognition.

In 1834 candidates for membership of the Royal College of Surgeons were examined by the whole Court of Examiners. By 1837 this was reduced to the less terrifying ordeal of facing three examiners only, and should there be any question of rejection a written examination was especially added for those whose results in the viva voce gave rise to doubt.

By 1838 the requirements had increased. Benjamin Brodie and Astley Cooper on behalf of the College wanted proof of a suitable preliminary education, three years' study in a recognised school of surgery, 21 months' work in hospital, dissection during two winter sessions, two six-month courses of lectures in anatomy, physiology and surgery, and one six-month course of lectures in chemistry, practical physic, midwifery, materia medica, and forensic medicine. The examiners (who were increased to four), still confined themselves to anatomy, physiology, surgery and surgical pathology.

It was a time when there was also a rise in the number of private medical schools in London such as the Webb Street School of Edward Grainger and the Aldersgate Street School of Frederick Tyrrell. Candidates seeking the LSA could attend these for tuition and also find their medical practice at dispensaries such as that of Aldersgate Street, founded in 1771 by John Coakley Lettsom, and entirely separate from the school of Tyrrell. Candidates seeking the MRCS in the 1820s were not required to have any formal instruction in 'physick'. They were not examined in midwifery, for which The Royal College of Surgeons did not institute any examination until 1852.

Not all apothecaries had a desire to practise pure medicine and certainly not all had a sense of professional decorum. Mapother records a placard noted in 1839 outside an apothecary's shop:

AB Surgeon and Apothecary. Prescriptions and family medicines accurately compounded. Teeth extracted at one shilling each. Women attended in labour 2s. 6d. each. Patent medicines and perfumery. Best London pickles. Fish sauces. Bear's grease. Soda water. Ginger Beer. Lemonade. Congreve matches, and Warren's blackening.

The proprietor confessed that he had no right to call himself a surgeon, but as a licentiate of the Society of Apothecaries he was legally qualified to practise medicine. These were not the men who were advancing the standards of general practice. Elsewhere the climate of opinion was encouraging improvement, although many general practitioners were hard pressed to find a living.

Arguments for keeping down the standards of examinations to maintain a supply of doctors willing to look after the poorer classes and work for local goverment medical services had to be strenuously opposed to achieve a single standard for medical practice. Sir Astley Cooper fittingly commented at a special BMA meeting of 1838, 'Let the guardians appoint those they would have for their own families, and they won't do wrong'.

HOSPITAL TEACHING

It is to be hoped that students in some places profited more from their hospital instruction than did Sir Robert Christison when a student at St Bartholomew's (figure 1) in the 1820s. He could not recollect 'having got a single useful lesson in the treatment of disease from the three physicians' there. Christison had lodged with Cullen in Well Yard, Little Britain, 'a puny row of students' lodging houses'. Cullen had been a surgical pupil at Bart's for six months and was 'well acquainted with Mr Lawrence, its Assistant Surgeon', a man who was Wakley's ardent supporter in the *Lancet* campaign for the College of Surgeons' reform. He had served for some time as prosector to Abernethy, who was at that time lecturer in anatomy and surgery to the hospital school.

Christison's destination, however, was medicine, not surgery. He was accordingly installed physician's pupil for a term of six months on payment of a fee of 16 guineas, but:

Alas for St Bartholomew's! The pupil found no teacher and found in the medical wards much more to teach others than for himself to learn.

At St Bartholomew's it was the rule that surgical students did not visit the medical wards unless duly entered as physician's pupils also, and it may be easily understood that few would purchase that privilege at the cost of sixteen guineas after expending the same sum on becoming pupils in the surgical department, but by use and wont physician's pupils were allowed freely into the surgical wards. . . .

The worst part of the hospital discipline at St Bartholomew's was the regulation (or rather non-regulation) of the pathological dissections. We had vast opportunities for following that branch of professional study, for many cases of organic diseases were admitted in their advanced stages. Mr Stanley, the anatomical demonstrator, was an ardent pathologist, and leave from the relatives of the deceased person was not, as in

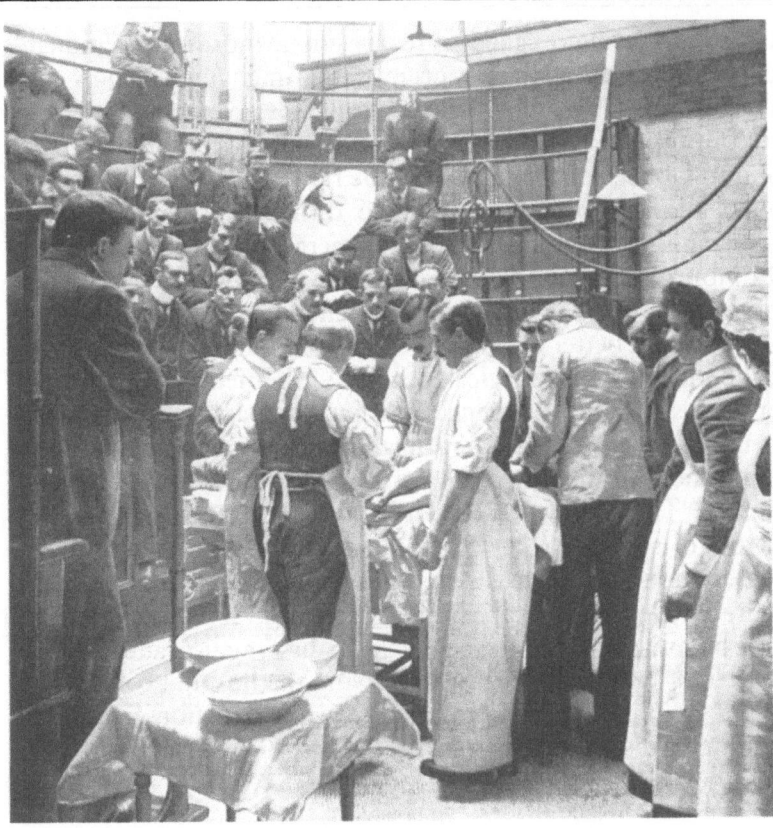

2. An operation at Charing Cross Hospital circa 1900.
Mary Evans Picture Library.

Edinburgh, a necessary condition. There was, therefore, usually a race between the relatives and the students, the former to carry off the body intact, the latter to dissect it. Thus dissection was apt to be performed with indecent, sometimes with dangerous haste. It was no uncommon occurrence that when the operator proceeded with his work the body was sensibly warm, the limbs not yet rigid, the blood in the great vessels fluid and coagulable.

Christison recalled an occasion when Cullen started the dissection of a man who had died suddenly, but one hour before. When fluid blood gushed in abundance from Cullen's first incision from top to bottom of the sternum, he seized his wrist in great alarm, 'Nor was I easily persuaded to let him go on when I saw the blood coagulate on the table exactly like living blood'. He preferred the system at Edinburgh where 24 hours had to elapse before autopsies were permitted.

Christison did not have a good opinion of the teaching at Bart's. It was a frequent source of wonder to him 'that so little use was made of the medical wards of St Bartholomew's for the purpose of instruction, and generally that education in medicine proper was almost entirely neglected'. While the medical students were only three in number and were allowed freely into the medical and surgical wards, the surgical students, amounting to several hundreds, never entered a medical ward. Yet the medical 'pupils', as they were called, in reality got no more information in medical practice than the few crumbs they might pick up now and then during the treatment of surgical cases. Nevertheless, men with only this training were passed annually in hundreds by the London College of Surgeons into the ranks of the general practitioners of England'. He found no difficulty in subsequently understanding the superiority of the general practitioners educated at Edinburgh. These were the men who were now excluded by the Apothecaries Act from practising as general practitioners.

He thought better of the surgical instruction received 'through the liberality of the surgical officers'; Abernethy and Vincent were the surgeons, Lawrence and Earle the assistant surgeons. Abernethy lectured in a small amphitheatre, notorious even among the unfeeling medical students of that age for its lack of comfort, 'The seats were without rails, and therefore each ascending row of students received the knees of those above into their backs, while they thrust theirs into those of the sitters below' (figure 2). George Hurst heard him lecture in 1820, 'By the pupils of the hospital he was esteemed as the highest medical authority of the period, and each student on leaving the hospital considered himself as only second, having received instruction from that great man's discourses'.

Medical Reform

The principal struggle for medical reform was rightly centred around the problem of an adequate medical education for the practitioner who was to look after the health of the majority of the people. As a result of the Act of 1815 it became established that he would have to qualify as LSA and to be truly a general practitioner he should hold the MRCS as well, although he could practise on the strength of either qualification.

ANATOMY TEACHING

The compulsory studies and dissections in anatomy brought about an increased trade in bodies and with it the distasteful necessities of grave robbing and body snatching. As early as 1788, it had been held to be a misdemeanour to disinter a body for the purpose of dissection. The court said that common decency required that the practice should be stopped, and that the offence was cognisable in a criminal court as being 'highly indecent and *contra bonos mores*, at the bare idea alone of which nature revolted'. It was observed in reference to this case that the act done would have been one of a peculiarly indecent theft, if it had not been for the technical reason that a dead body is not the subject of property. It was the custom to try these malefactors at the Old Bailey. The public became so alarmed about the desecration of the dead that such inventions as Bridgeman's patent wrought iron coffin came into use to foil the grave snatchers. The employment of grave watchers was not unusual.

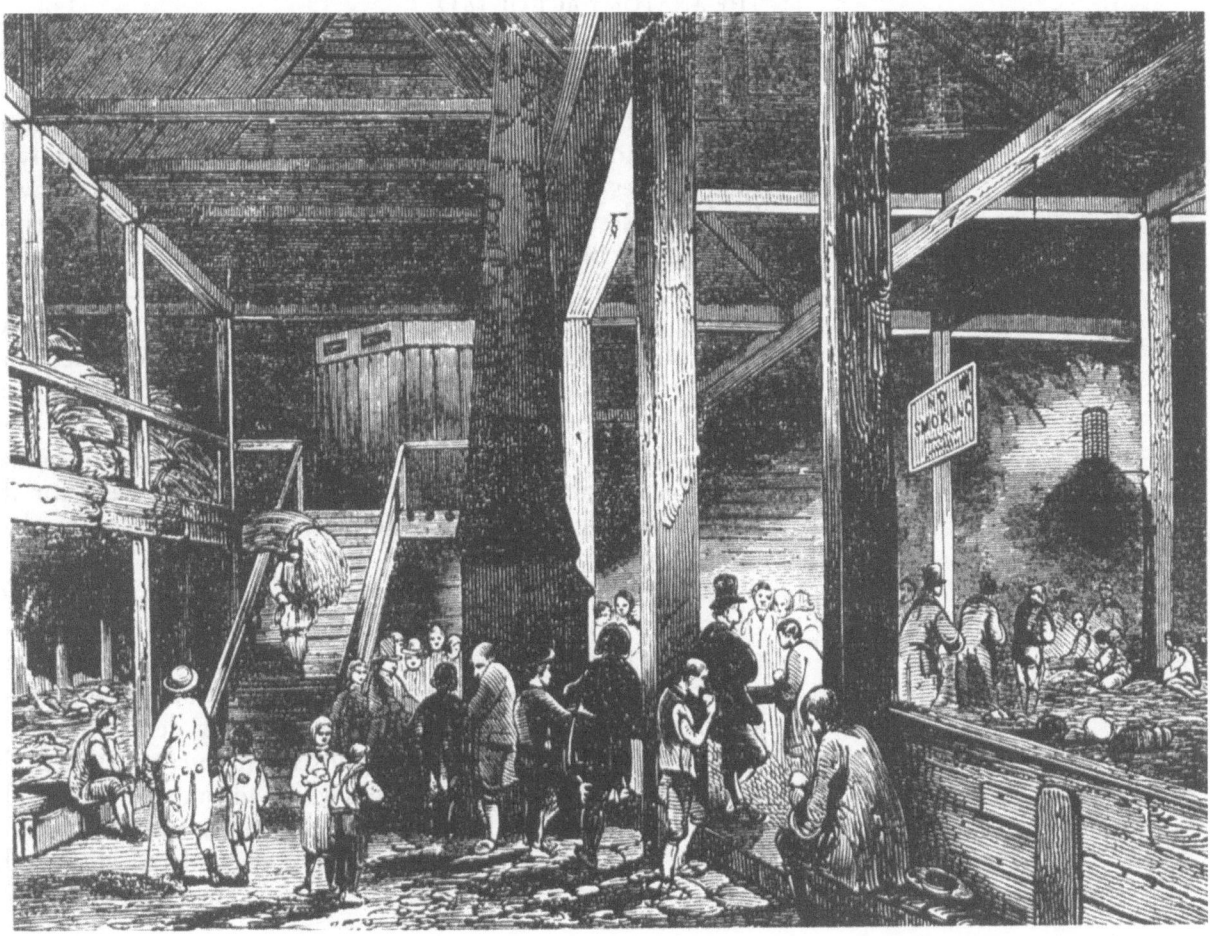

Matters, however, became much worse when murder was committed to maintain the supply of bodies. Robert Knox (1791–1862) was a disciple of Bichat and his anatomical lectures and demonstrations were a great attraction for students to come to Edinburgh to study. The trade in bodies there was good. On 29 November 1827, one William Hare conceived the notion that he would recover a debt of £4, owed him by a deceased tenant of his, by selling the old man's body. This he subsequently did for £7 10s to Robert Knox. Following this profitable transaction he formed an association with a man called Burke, and together they evolved the business practice of 'burking'. This involved making the victim drunk, and then suffocating him by closing the hands tightly over his nose and mouth. At least 16 people were murdered, and the tale is told of a beautiful girl whose body was recognised by medical students! Burke and Hare were apprehended. Another victim's body was found boxed up in Knox's rooms and public anger mounted against him ruined his career. The outcry benefited anatomy in bringing home to Parliament that a supply of cadavers for dissection was necessary. Burke's body was fittingly handed over after execution for anatomising, while Hare escaped this fate by turning King's evidence.

3. Refuge for the destitute; the male ward of a Poor House, circa 1840. *BBC Hulton Picture Library.*

THE ANATOMY ACT OF 1832

The Anatomy Act of 1832 recites the importance of anatomy and recognises that 'the legal supply of human bodies for such anatomical examination is insufficient fully to provide the means of such knowledge'. It then makes provision for the supply of such bodies by enabling 'any executor or other party having lawful possession of the body of any deceased person' to permit the body to be dissected, except in special cases. The effect was that the bodies of persons dying in various public institutions (figure 3), whose relatives were unknown, were given up for dissection. It also enacted that after examination, the bodies 'shall be decently interred'. This Act showed clearly that Parliament regarded anatomical dissection as a legal practice and, furthermore, that there was such a thing as 'a legal supply of human bodies', though until then there had been insufficient for the purpose. Medical education had received a considerable mark of recognition.

The development of a general medical service for the people of this country, with an adequate number of professionally qualified general practitioners, was eventually made possible by the determination of the medical rank and file to ensure an acceptable standard of education. Despite its inherent deficiencies, the Apothecaries Act of 1815, by its subsequent interpretation in the courts, was the rallying point from which advance was made. The movement for medical reform was born and nurtured within the medical profession. The enthusiasm it engendered created the favourable climate of opinion which was to ensure its success.

Reform of the Medical Profession

After the accession of Queen Victoria to the throne, there were in her realm no fewer than 21 portals of entry to the medical profession via 11 universities, 9 medical corporations and the Archbishop of Canterbury! Yet they did not all have the power to give an unlimited right to practise medicine and surgery anywhere in Great Britain and Ireland. This privilege was still reserved for the Royal College of Physicians, and the universities of Oxford or Cambridge, by courtesy. Only Dublin could exclude the old elite, for in that city the King and Queen's College of Physicians had the sole rights over licences to practise medicine. The Apothecaries Act had brought home to Scottish and Irish graduates that they could no longer practise in England and Wales without licence of the London Apothecaries. The Society of Apothecaries, since the 1815 Act, had *de jure* if not *de facto* control of general practice in England and Wales; at least in so far as it was conducted by people calling themselves apothecaries.

THE NEED FOR REFORM

The Apothecaries Act did not define an apothecary although it referred to apothecarial and not to medical practice. One of its immediate effects was to prevent the medical practitioner from dispensing unless he was prepared to undergo the five-year apprenticeship necessary before taking the apothecaries' examination. This was a serious handicap to all medical graduates from the Scottish, Irish and foreign universities together with provincial English graduates and all surgeons.

In Scotland the Faculty of Physicians and Surgeons of Glasgow only held the licensing power over Lanark, Renfrew, Ayr, Burgh and Dumbarton; the Royal College of Surgeons of Edinburgh had the monopoly of the Three Lothians, Fife, Roxburgh, Berwick, Selkirk and Peebles. The Edinburgh College of Physicians had defined powers in and around Edinburgh. The Worshipful Society of Apothecaries of Dublin had similar powers to its London counterpart, while members of each required the licence of the other to practise in its territory. In Ireland, outside Dublin, graduates in physic of Oxford, Cambridge, London and Dublin were allowed to practise without the specific licence of the King and Queen's College of Physicians. This was about the only privilege that London graduates could boast. Neither they nor Durham graduates by virtue of their medical degrees had the right to practise in their own capital city of London. It was thus no easy matter for the public to recognise a safely qualified doctor, for he who was acceptable in Bideford or Tipperary was not necessarily recognised in Wapping.

The overall standard of medical education had improved by the middle of the eighteenth century and the profession as a whole had a greater pride throughout its ranks, although there were considerable variations still in standard between one qualifying body and the next. The demands for improvement were coming from within the profession and were attained partly through the interaction of various medical societies and their leaders, and with John Simon as a sort of *eminence grise* (figure 1).

MEDICAL ASSOCIATIONS

The nineteenth century saw the burgeoning of medical societies, which grouped practitioners together for all sorts of medical, social and political reasons. They were often forums for scientific discussions. The medico-political associations were primarily interested in medical education and standards of care, and the status of the doctor. The Worcester Medical and Surgical Society founded by Charles Hastings in 1816 had had a hand in the

1. Sir John Simon (1816–1904). Lithograph by C. Baugniet. In the Wellcome Institute. *By courtesy of the Wellcome Trustees.*

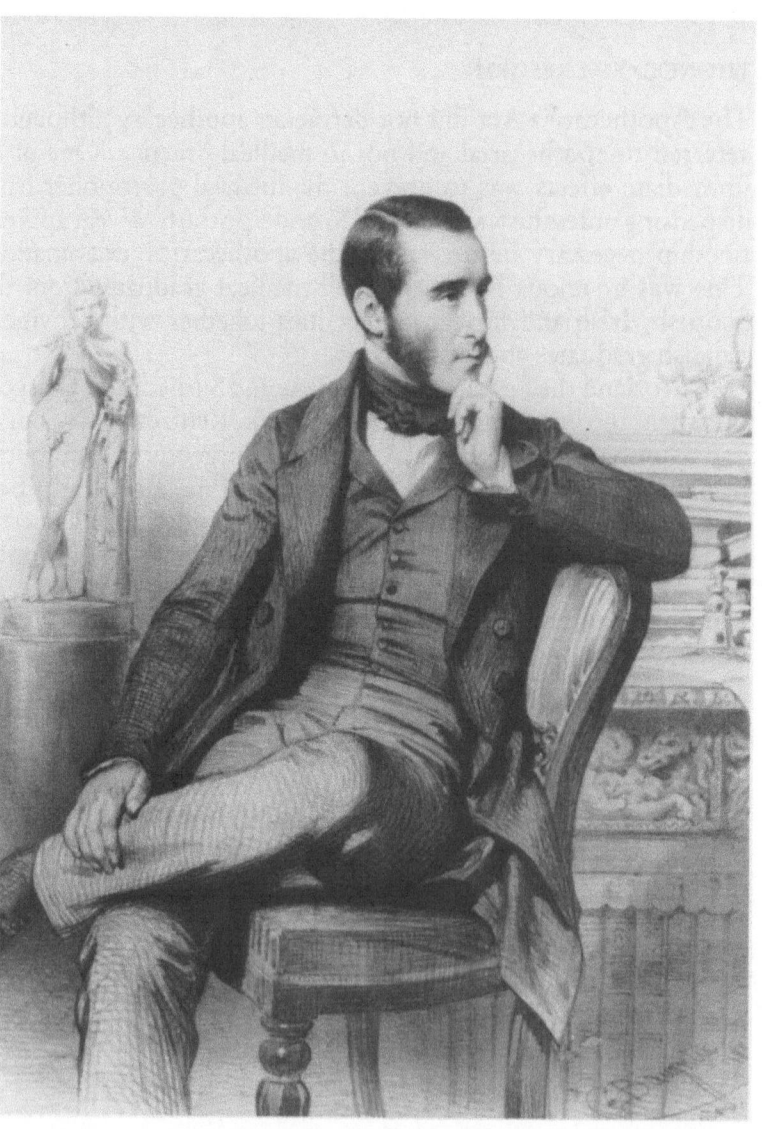

Anatomy Bill of 1828, enacted in 1832.

Various societies were formed by general practitioners, who now represented the largest part of the profession. John Bellers had referred to this group as 'general Practitioners in Physick' in his *Essay Towards the Improvement of Physick* of 1714. The term general practitioner was not in common use in the early nineteenth century. William Gaitskell founded the Metropolitan Society of General Practitioners in 1830. Thomas Wakley, editor of *The Lancet*, showed his vehement dislike for the use of 'general practitioner' in the title and the Society did not last long. The Association of Apothecaries and Surgeon-Apothecaries was reorganised to form the Association of General Practitioners of England and Wales in 1833, on the occasion of the Apothecaries Act Amendment Bill.

The Provincial Medical and Surgical Association was founded at Worcester by Charles Hastings in 1832, for physicians, surgeons and general practitioners and took over his journal, *The Midland Medical and Surgical Reporter*. Wakley at first approved of this society, but objected to the provincial title Hastings had given it. However, it was not until 23 years later that it became known as the British Medical Association. He also furiously protested that the Association had become orientated towards the consultant at the expense of the ordinary practitioner.

2. The General Infirmary at Leeds in 1771.
Reproduced by permission of S. T. Anning, from The Apothecaries of the General Infirmary at Leeds.

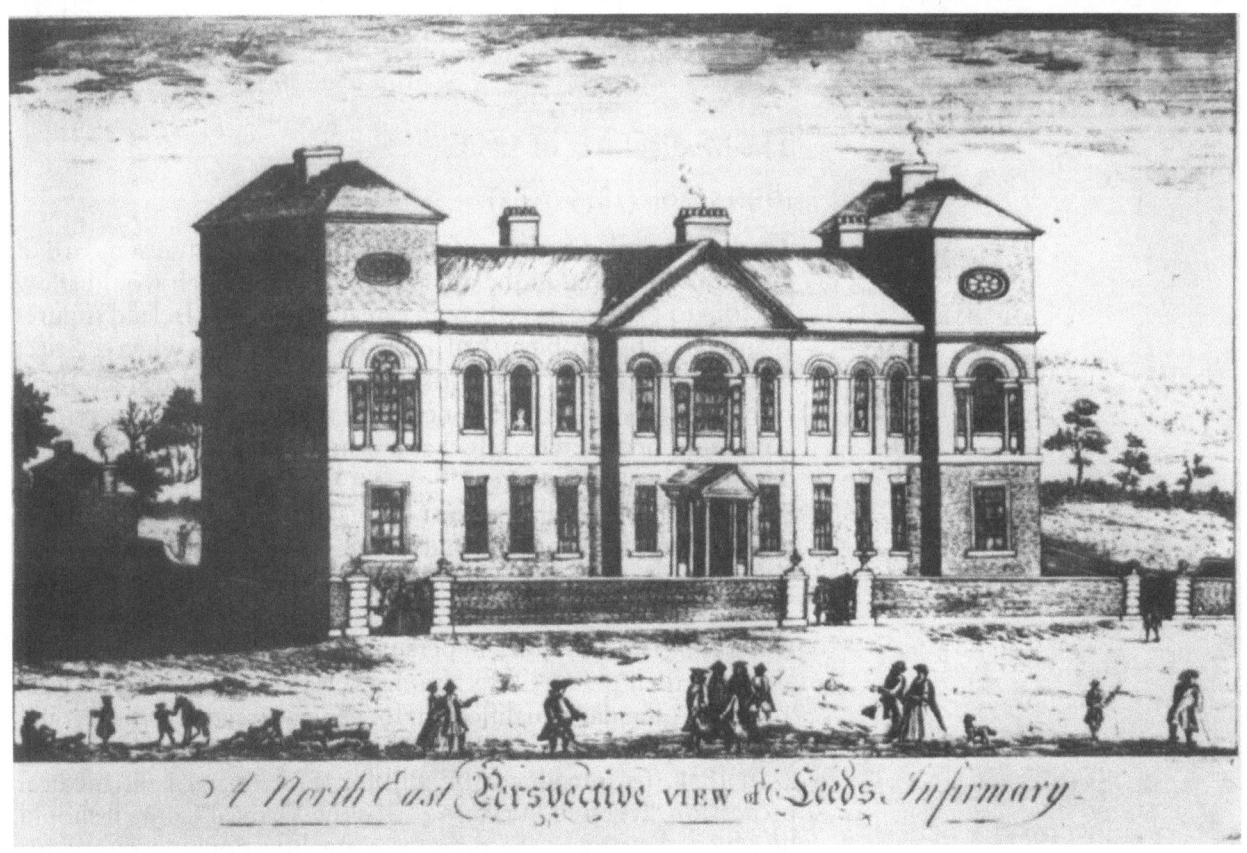

Some members of the profession wished to put general practitioners under the control of the Royal College of Surgeons, with which they felt they had the closest historical links. Even today, this connection is shown in the use of the word 'surgery' for the general practitioner's consulting room. The group supporting this move united to form the National Association of General Practitioners, which later became the National Institute of General Practitioners. Wakley supported this group, until it changed its mind about joining the surgeons and began agitating for a new college for general practitioners. W. Robins also opposed this move in a letter to *The Lancet* in 1848:

The voice of the intellectual world had declared the science of medicine to be a whole—divisible into parts in practice solely for utility and convenience—but it had not declared that for the proper application of this science a new college is needed.
If advancement to its Inner Temple of Fame cannot be insured without the stimulus of other rewards, than those invariably accompanying merit, let them be offered—but no attempt be made to cripple merit by the false glare of inferior colleges, or by promulgating to the world false notions of real worth.

These medical associations played a not inconsiderable part in the legislation which affected the development of general practice, the Poor Law Amendment Act of 1834, the Births and Deaths Registration Act of 1836, the Vaccination Act of 1840 and the Public Health Act of 1848.

The Medical Act of 1858

JOHN SIMON (1816–1904)

There was a need for some form of overall minimum standard of education required in the medical profession which would allow doctors to practise anywhere in Great Britain and Ireland (figures 2 and 3). The problem had been raised in 1834 when a Select Committee was formed to look into the matter, and again in 1847. However, any reform was once again thwarted by the three main governing bodies who felt that a central medical council would diminish their own power.

John Simon, medical officer to the General Board of Health, was determined to bring about a 'one portal' entry to the profession and he used all his power, plus a few anonymous letters to *The Times*, in his attempts to achieve this. He realised that there would be great difficulty in persuading the 21 licensing bodies to abrogate their powers. His aim, however, was to establish a legal 'minimum standard qualification for general practice', which could later be supplemented by higher degrees and diplomas.

In 1858, he introduced his Bill for the reform of the medical profession. It stated in clause 4, that the Medical Council should be given the power 'to define the qualifications necessary for registration, to allow or disallow the certificates of the various medical bodies as evidence of qualification, to compel these bodies to combine into conjoint examination boards, and to conduct its own examinations if those provided elsewhere were unsatisfactory'. Clause 4 did not get into the Act.

The Medical Act of 1858 achieved certain fundamental advances. It created a central professional governing body, it gave the right to the legally qualified practitioner to practise throughout the realm, and it made a register of practitioners which the public could recognise. The newly created General Council of Medical Education and Registration was at first more than a little over-awed by the multiplicity of 'competitive licence-mongering bodies'.

Simon had not achieved the power he had hoped for; thwarted and frustrated he violated his own 'one portal' principle by creating special qualifications for vaccination! With skill and tenacity of purpose, John Simon then used his Presidency of the Medical Teachers' Association, which he had accepted in 1867, to press on with his 'one portal' ideas. Adroitly managing the Royal College of Surgeons, he forced the Medical Council to consider the need for a single minimum qualification and a consolidated examination authority. The Medical Act (1858) Amendment Bill intended that conjoint examination boards should be set up in England and Wales, Scotland and Ireland. Candidates accepted for the new diploma of 'licentiate in medicine and surgery' were to be registered and thus the 'one portal' entry would have been achieved. Despite a carefully prepared climate of public and professional opinion, the Bill foundered in 1870 on the issue of the representation of general practitioners on the Medical Council. Neither did the profession care for the powers given in the Bill for the Privy

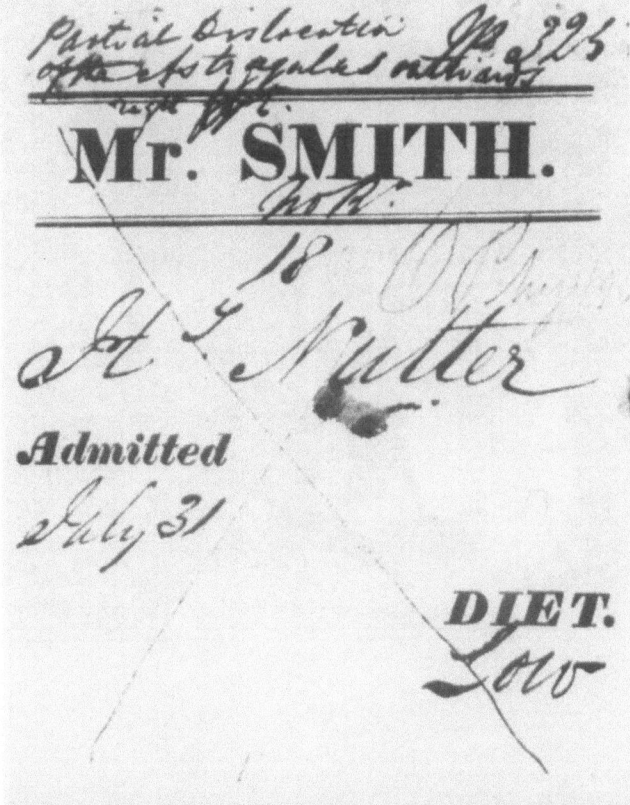

3. A bed ticket for a patient admitted to the General Infirmary at Leeds, in July 1831. Reproduced from *Medical History*, 1961, Volume 5. *By courtesy of the Wellcome Trustees.*

Council to modify or confirm examination conditions at its discretion, even to the extent of dissolving examination boards. John Simon was seen as a possible medical dictator, but even a dictator with the highest motives and abilities was unacceptable.

THE CONJOINT DIPLOMA

All practitioners who had passed either the LSA or MRCS were allowed to register, following the 1858 Act, but both examinations were deficient in certain areas. This deficiency indicated the desirability of a common conjoint diploma. In 1859, the College of Surgeons suggested that it should join the College of Physicians to produce a joint examination. The General Medical Council did not approve this conjoint diploma MRCS (Eng) LRCP (Lond) until 1884. In the interim, therefore, the College of Surgeons modified its own MRCS, making it a comprehensive examination of surgery, medicine and midwifery. The new conjoint diploma

4. A 'street doctor' in 1870, selling cough lozenges.
BBC Hulton Picture Library.

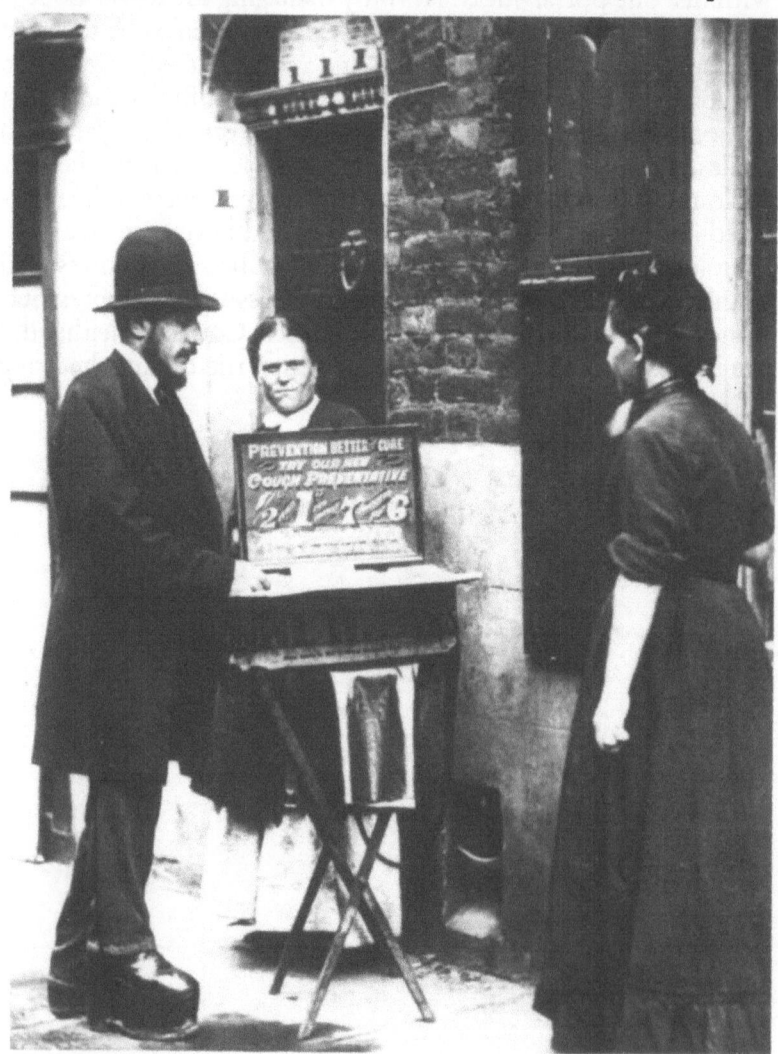

superseded it to become the recognised qualification for general practitioners, for the next 50 years. It provided a new portal of entry into the profession, but not the 'one portal' for which many of the reformers had hoped. Many still took a university degree alone or in addition to the diploma.

UNQUALIFIED PRACTITIONERS

Despite the 1858 Act, there were still many unqualified practitioners. The 40th clause of the Act stated:

Any person who shall wilfully and falsely pretend to be, or take or use the name or title of a Physician, Doctor of Medicine, Licentiate in Medicine and Surgery, Bachelor of Medicine, Surgeon, General Practitioner or Apothecary, or any name, title, addition or description implying that he is registered under this Act, or that he is recognised by law as a Physician or Surgeon, or Licentiate in Medicine and Surgery, or a Practitioner in Medicine, or an Apothecary, shall upon summary conviction for any such offence pay a sum not exceeding twenty pounds.

This clause could not be used against those who had never pretended to be registered. There were still many people who were quite happy to be treated by unregistered practitioners, particu-

5. An advertisement in 1891 for the Carbolic Smoke Ball, claiming it will cure a variety of ailments from 'headache' to 'throat deafness'. *BBC Hulton Picture Library.*

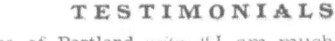
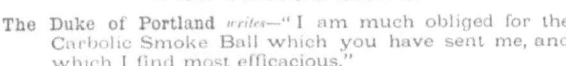

CARBOLIC SMOKE BALL

WILL POSITIVELY CURE

COUGHS	BRONCHITIS	INFLUENZA	NEURALGIA
COLDS	THROAT DEAFNESS	SORE THROAT	WHOOPING
CATARRH	HOARSENESS	HAY FEVER	COUGH
ASTHMA	LOSS OF VOICE	CROUP	HEADACHE

As all the Diseases mentioned above proceed from one cause, they can be CURED by one remedy, viz

The **CARBOLIC SMOKE BALL.** As prescribed by **SIR MORELL MACKENZIE, M D.,** and other eminent **Physicians.**

TESTIMONIALS.

The Duke of Portland *writes*—"I am much obliged for the Carbolic Smoke Ball which you have sent me, and which I find most efficacious."

The Bishop of London *writes*—"The Carbolic Smoke Ball has benefited me greatly."

Lady Mostyn *writes*—"Lady Mostyn believes the Carbolic Smoke Ball to be a certain check and cure for a cold."

Lady Erskine *writes*—"The Carbolic Smoke Ball has given every satisfaction."

Lady Clavering *writes*—"The Carbolic Smoke Ball has been invaluable to her daughter."

Lady Feilden *writes*—"Lady Feilden is always glad to recommend the Smoke Ball, as it is most efficacious."

Mrs. Gladstone *writes*—"She finds the Carbolic Smoke Ball has done her a great deal of good."

One CARBOLIC SMOKE BALL will last a family several months, making it the Cheapest Remedy in the world at the price—**10s.**, Post Free.

The CARBOLIC SMOKE BALL can be refilled when empty at a cost of 5s., Post Free.

ADDRESS:

CARBOLIC SMOKE BALL CO., 27, PRINCES ST., HANOVER SQ., LONDON, W.

larly as even those doctors who had been formally educated could do little when faced with serious disease (figures 4 and 5). The unqualified practitioners were given encouragement by Lord Chief Justice Cockburn when he ruled in favour of Hamilton, the 'anti-registered botanic surgeon'. The judge decided that there was 'nothing in the Act to prevent a person from merely practising as a surgeon without being registered'.

Rivington, in his book *The Medical Profession*, quotes from a coroner's inquest of 1875 in which Mr Bigwood, an unqualified herbalist, had to defend the death of his patient. His evidence shows how little some medical practice and beliefs in the lower classes, had changed from the Middle Ages:

I am a 'licensed botanist', residing at Corsham. I was first requested to visit the deceased on May 11th. He was then downstairs sitting in a chair. I told him I thought I might, but it would be like raising the dead from the grave; but the deceased wished me to give him a trial. I then asked him if he was under a doctor. He said 'Yes, but the doctor says he can do no more for me'. I told him I would give him a trial; but I did not think I should raise him, for he had no blood in him. I told him that his liver did not throw any blood . . . as he looked as sallow as death. I sent him a bottle of medicine next day which contained seven different sorts of herbs. They were herbs governed by the sun. These herbs strengthen the heart, which I wished to do.

6. Wandsworth School Treatment Centre.
The Greater London Council Photographic Library.

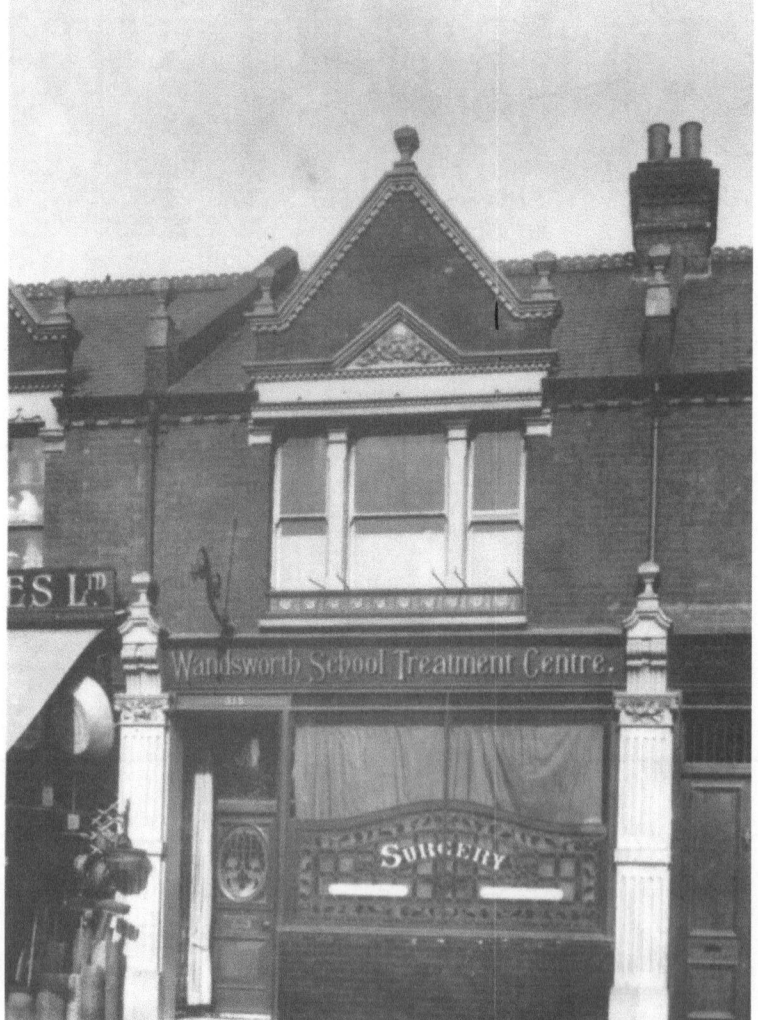

I work on a botanist scale of astrology. I send medicine all over the country. I consider that my licence allows me to do so. When I advertise I advertise for fits. I do not advertise for consumption, for I know it is no good. I use a hundred different sorts of herbs. I give medicine for every part of the body where it is afflicted. I use the Government stamp on all bottles of medicine sent out, no matter what are the contents.

The medicine I gave him was for the chest, heart, lungs, and liver. I sent him 4 bottles of medicine and a box of 20 pills—the pills to be taken with the medicine. The pills were made with the same herbs as the mixture, ground into powder with cayenne, hickory-picry, and rhubarb ... I ask for hickory-picry, for I know no other name for it. I have raised men very near from the grave with that medicine and pills. I have been practising 12 years. I judge all complaints by astronomy. If I have the date of a man's birth, if he lived in London and sent to Corsham to tell me he was bad, I could tell what his complaint was, and what to prescribe for him. This I have done many times and made many cures. The deceased was born on 6 January 1852 (I do not know the hour and minute). The sun was in opposition sign with the stomach when he was born; that showed that the sun stood in afflicted sign to the body. The moon rules the liver, and that is where his disease was, and that is what he died from. I never had a patient die that had been taking my medicine since I have been in practice. If they fall worse, I tell them they must get a doctor. By watching the movements of the heavens I can tell when to call in an experimental medical man, or there would be many such caddies as this, as I would not be responsible for their lives unto the end without further counsel — I would not be responsible as there would be upsets about it. I do not confine women or do bone-setting.

The jury returned a verdict of death from natural causes, but stated that he was lucky not to be committed to Gloucester jail on a charge of manslaughter. Mr Bigwood, however, had been careful not to offend the 1858 Act, and could not be charged under section 40 as he had never claimed to be registered.

General Practitioners

DIFFERENT TYPES OF GENERAL PRACTITIONERS

Rivington divided the general practitioners into 'dispensing and non-dispensing orders'. In the dispensing order he subdivided them into two suborders: '(a) The surgeon-chemist, or the red-bottle and blue-bottle practitioners, who combine the work of medical men with the retail business of a chemist'. These men kept shops, with glass cases full of tooth brushes, nail brushes, patent medicines, fruit salts, soaps and feeding bottles. They depended primarily on retail trade. The next suborder was '(b) The surgeon-apothecary, with an open surgery and a red lamp.' No retail trade was done here, and usually a shilling was charged for advice and a bottle of medicine. Some of these men kept dispensaries and attended patients for a weekly sum of 2d to 1s. As the social scale was ascended the surgery of the surgeon-apothecary receded from the front window type (figure 6) into the interior 'no longer exposed to the vulgar gaze'. If it succeeded in disappearing entirely it qualified for the non-dispensing or consultant order. Medicines prescribed were made up at the chemist's and patients were seen and visited at lower fees than those of the pures or regular physicians. All these groups of general practitioners shaded off one into the other.

THE WORK OF THE GENERAL PRACTITIONER

In 1890, Jukes De Styrap published *The Young Practitioner: with practical hints and instructive suggestions—as subsidiary aids—for his guidance on entering into Private Practice*. This book gives a very idealised picture of the Victorian general practitioner, but it does provide an insight into his role and work.

De Styrap did not recommend working partnerships:

The partners are not, as a rule, equally matched in industry, capacity for professional work, temperament, tact, and other essential qualities, indispensable to a congenial and intimate fellowship.

He felt that a co-partnership could work for a limited period 'with an elderly practitioner desirous to retire'.

He stated that a great deal of care should be taken in the selection of premises: they should be 'in a good and comparatively retired neighbourhood', with a recessed or private entrance as 'patients in general have an aversion to be seen standing at the doctor's'. He added:

7. Dr John Owen Jones with his chauffeur, outside his surgery about to set off on his rounds. The building is still a surgery.
By courtesy of Dr J. G. Thomas.

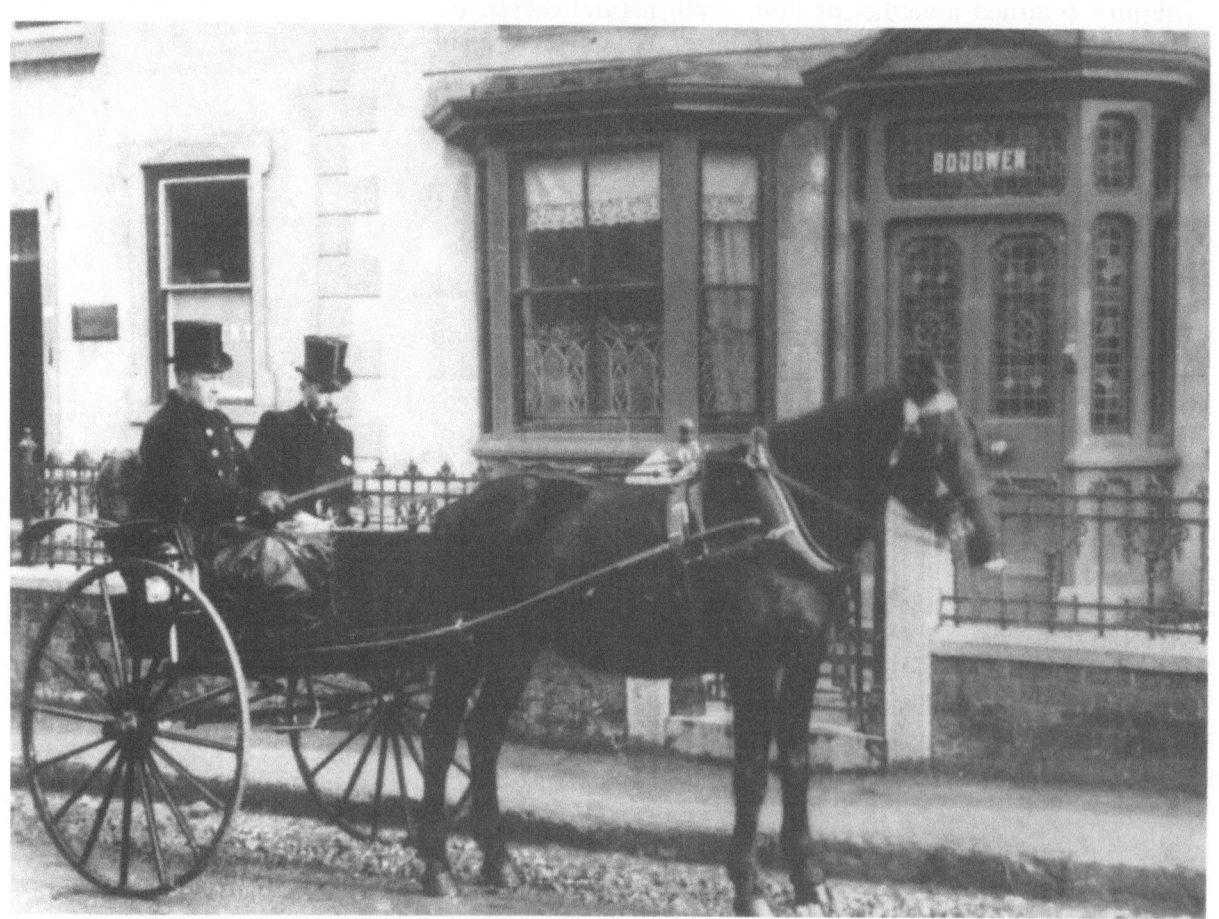

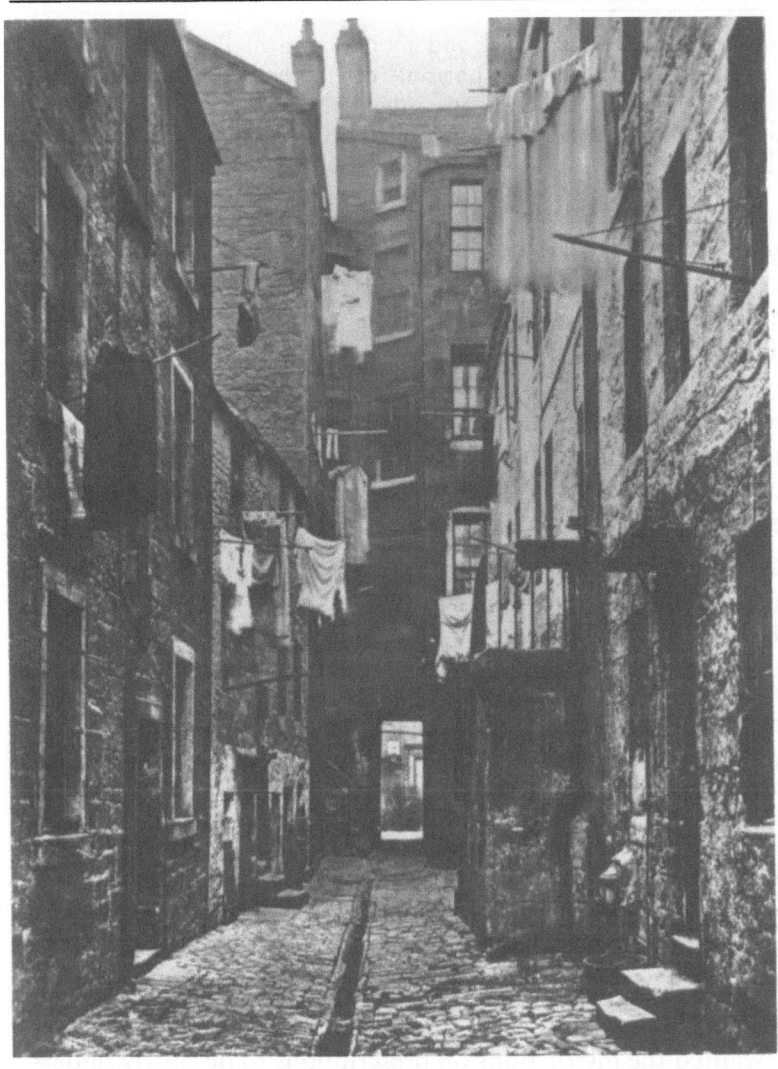

8. A Glasgow tenement during the mid
nineteenth century.
Mansell Collection.

In regard to your doorplate, let it be of strictly moderate dimensions,
and the name well and distinctly engraved; . . . When entitled thereto, it
is better to put Dr . . ., than . . ., MD. The former not only looks best,
but has the advantage of being understood by all classes. As a representative title of the 'General Practitioner', so termed, personally I entertain
a predilection for the old familiar one of 'Surgeon', in preference to that
of modern innovation—Physician and Surgeon'.

His book gives instructions about the arrangement of the
surgery. He advised that 'repelling objects' such as syringes,
specula and gynaecological couch, should be relegated to 'the
dark corner of the room', and even advised against the display of
'framed and glazed diplomas of proficiency in anatomy and
kindred sciences'. Articles which should be given prominence
included:

microscope, stethoscope, laryngoscope, ophthalmoscope, urinary
cabinet (one designed by the author and manufactured by Messrs Maw,

London, will be found useful, and not unornamental) and other aids to precision in diagnosis, with portraits of eminent professional friends and teachers, and academical and other prizes denotive of the mental and physical prowess which distinguished the young practitioner in his still earlier days . . .

Certain instruments should be taken on the doctor's professional rounds (figure 7), in a 'neat pocket case': a clinical thermometer, female catheter, bistoury, small forceps, hypodermic syringe, lunar caustic, probe and needles.

De Styrap felt that it was relatively easy to find work among the moneyless poor but more difficult with the upper class. It was, however, by treating the wealthy classes that a doctor could build his reputation although he had to beware of becoming known as the doctor who looked after the servants. He offered advice on the doctor's personal conduct:

In cases of danger, or other pressing necessity, you need not hesitate to undertake any menial work for a patient; but unless such cause exists, to pull off your coat, administer an injection, give a bath, swaddle a new-born babe, rummage drawers or ransack cupboards in search of towels, old linen for bandages, spoons, goblets, etc will ill-comport with your position, and may be quoted against you as evincing a sad lack of professional dignity and self respect. It is far better to ask for the things you need, and let them be brought to you.

The book includes useful tips on how to deal with common problems:

It may be important to you to remember that, contrary to the popular belief, the art of medicine does not enable you, or any other practitioner to diagnose positively any of the eruptive fevers, until their local manifestations appear.

He wanted the instructions on prescriptions to be clearly understood and recommended that they should be in English and that the times for taking the medicine should be given by the clock rather than simply 'four hourly'. The doctor should take care 'never to prescribe a proprietary remedy, or one covered by a trade-mark'.

De Styrap relied on the recommendations of the British Medical Association for medico-chirurgical tariffs. This stated that patients should pay medical fees proportional to the rental value of their houses, but this system should also be adjusted to make it 'a fair and equitable remuneration, accordant with the patient's position and ability to pay' (figure 8). De Styrap added that doctors should charge their patients according to the value of their time and skill, 'and altogether ignore the objectionable system of "drug payment".'

Specialisation

The Medical Act of 1858 had led to a minimum standard of medical education being laid down for the qualification of the 'safe doctor'. It was a standard motivated by the manifest need of the profession and the public for a general medical practitioner who could be recognised as competent. Once legally qualified, he was to be able to practise anywhere within the United Kingdom and perform any medical or surgical treatment without further qualification, or indeed further training. This gave rise to a convenient, in many ways desirable and unquestionably unifying fiction that all doctors were equal in the sight of man and of the law. In the higher echelons of Society, equality in the sight of man had never followed from the long accepted tenet of equality under the law. The latest entrants to the profession hoped that this equality under the law would lead to an elevation of their social status, whilst the older physicians feared that it would lower theirs. Although these distinctions were in the course of time to become increasingly blurred, the methods of qualification leading to registration still continued to distinguish the university graduate, and particularly those of Oxford and Cambridge, for a further century.

In the 'new' profession, most doctors also continued to practise from their own homes, where social distinctions were again most easily recognisable. Moreover, the increasing population and the development of hospitals meant that yet another distinction within the profession was about to flourish as the numbers and prestige of the hospital doctors grew.

GROWTH OF SPECIALISATION

With the increase of knowledge in medicine came the realisation that the original idea of registration for a safely qualified general practitioner would have in time to be modified to allow the alternative of a safely qualified specialist.

William Osler recognised the increasing importance of specialisation in his lifetime. Even in 1892 he was able to say, 'The rapid increase of knowledge has made concentration of work a necessity; specialism is here and here to stay'. The word itself had not been used in its modern sense before 1856, though of course healers may have had their special interests from very early days. In Wales there was the example of the bonesetters of Anglesey, whose skills were passed on to the father of orthopaedic surgery, Hugh Owen Thomas. Specialism was slow to achieve respectability and even today the veterinary profession does not look kindly upon claims to specialisation.

For a specialist to succeed he must not only have the special knowledge, but he must be able to draw on a large pool of patients. The conditions which make this possible are of good communications to spread his fame and reliable travel facilities to reach him. Newspapers and improved road, rail and sea passages of the nineteenth century, which themselves had grown out of increased knowledge of the sciences, catalysed the process. Few British towns had a population large enough to encourage much more specialisation than that between physician and surgeon.

The general practitioners and the physicians of that age were problem solvers. With laboratory medicine in its childhood, and only limited ancillary aids to narrow diagnosis, clinical problems were presented to these men, whose function was to produce an hypothesis to fit the signs and symptoms. The fame of these skilful clinicians rested on their ability to find and interpret clues which could lead to classification of illness. In the nineteenth century, and even into the twentieth, one great man was expected

1. William Osler on the ward. This photograph was taken by C. E. Brush and is from the Johns Hopkins Hospital Album 1903–1904.
By courtesy of the Osler Library, Montreal.

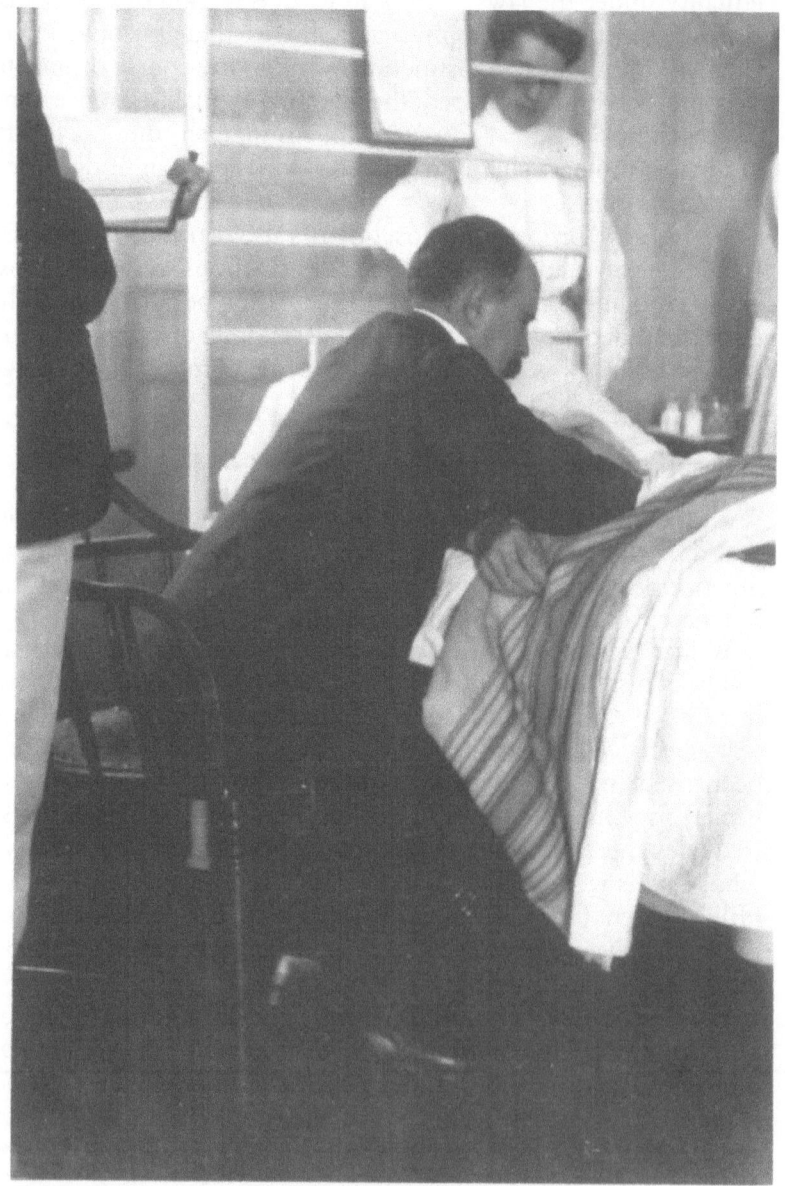

to do this and to do it alone. No single doctor can ever again be so omniscient. In the late twentieth century he has been replaced by a team of specialists who pool the results, a sort of diagnosis by committee, but still requiring the practical judgement of a clinician to initiate and manage treatment.

SPECIALIST OR CONSULTANT

In his address to the fourth annual meeting of the Paediatric Society at Boston in 1892, Osler (figure 1) thanked the Society for:

Choosing as your presiding officer one whose work has lain in the wide field of general medicine which is an indication that you duly appreciate the relation of the special subject in which we are now interested, and to which this society is devoted. The diseases incident to infancy and childhood are so varied, covering every department of internal medicine, as well as of surgery, that the broad distinctions emphasised by the names physician and surgeon suffice to characterise us, and happily we have not as yet been stamped with a distinctive appellation, under which so many of our colleagues in other lines labour.

At that time, the word paediatrician was not in common use.

Already in the larger cities, the work of the specialist was encroaching on that of the general practitioner, and Osler said:

This condition, though in many ways to be regretted, is not likely to be changed. I have known the head of a household pay, in the course of a year, for the professional services of six physicians—a gynaecologist, an oculist, a laryngologist, a dermatologist, and a surgeon. What remained after this partition, the general practitioner, came in sixth and looked after the health of the children.

It is interesting to note that to this one pertains the functions to a large extent of the old family doctor, and further advice is usually sought through him or at his suggestion. In the evolution of the specialist the children's doctor is the last to appear, not because of any extreme differentiation, but rather he is the vestigial remnant of what was formerly in cities the general practitioner.

He was, of course talking of the USA, where the process started earlier and eventually developed farther than has the attrition of the general practitioner in Britain, but his observations were of universal import. The geriatrician has appeared since Osler's time and now leaves the general practitioner with less of a life span than ever to look after. It would not be too surprising, with the urgent problems associated with transplants, to find the emergence of mortologists or death specialists.

At first, not many of the better qualified doctors of the 'old school' were specialists. Many continued their traditional distinction from the apothecaries and maintained their generic status as consultants. The new equality of professional rights under the law had led to an interesting reversal of the bases for financial competition. No longer was it the physician who complained that the apothecary was diminishing his income by treating the patient directly, without his referral. It was now the general practitioner who complained that the consultant was seeing his patient, without any professional request, and then compounding the offence by continuing to treat him and collect the fees.

Threats to general practice in the USA in 1892 became a *fait accompli* there in the twentieth century. This did not happen in Britain where the College of General Practitioners was founded in 1952, just over a century since a previous attempt had failed.

2. Complaints which appeared in the *British Medical Journal*. 1. 23 July 1892. 2. 18 February 1893. *By courtesy of the British Medical Journal.*

CASUALTY PATIENTS AT ST. BARTHOLOMEW'S

"The annual statement of the clerk of St. Bartholomew's Hospital states that 5,953 in-patients, 16,143 out-patients, and 142,745 casualty patients were treated there during the year." We would call the serious attention of all those interested in hospital reform—and this includes the whole medical profession as well as a large proportion of the lay public—to the course pursued at St. Bartholomew's. The abuses of the out-patient system have been demonstrated till the very fulness of proof has produced satiety, and the subject is voted stale. No one denies them: but by calling one class of out-patients "casualties" (which they are not in any sense beyond the most insignificant fraction of the number), an attempt is being made to perpetuate and even aggravate the evils of the system.

In the out-patient department some inquiry is possible, both into the patient's circumstances and the nature of the case; treatment can be deliberate and efficacious, clinical teaching may be carried out. But think of 140,000 persons jostling through the casualty room in a single year! Investigation is precluded, treatment is a farce, teaching is not even professed. And yet, in spite of the universal public opinion, both of the lay and medical public, this system, of which we cannot trust ourselves to write in the terms it deserves, is kept up at the very hospital where it was so mercilessly exposed to public scorn and reprobation by one of the casualty physicians themselves—Dr. R. Bridges in the *St. Batholomew's Hospital Reports*—and under the implied sanction of medical men high in office at the Colleges of Physicians and Surgeons.

MEDICAL AND ASSOCIATIONS

Another Sufferer writes: I can fully endorse all your correspondent "One of Them" says about the above named associations, and can myself speak with some authority on the subject, having acted as medical officer to one of the so called friendly societies' medical aid associations for about six months, at the end of which time I threw up the appointment in disgust. The subscription, entitling a man, his wife, and all members of his family under 16 years of age to professional attendance and medicines was 2s. 6d. a quarter, and it was surprising to me the number of exceedingly well to do individuals I had to attend for that sum—people, judging from their surroundings and the manner in which they lived, perfectly able to pay the usual fees for medical advice. I will say nothing about being kept "on the trot" from morning till night attending to ailments of an absurdly trivial nature. (I was once called up at night to see a woman two miles from the house who had got the toothache.) But I did object to have to pull teeth out at 3d. a time from the jaws of those quite in a position to pay 2s. 6d. to the dentist.

Hospitals and the General Practitioner

Until the beginning of the nineteenth century, most medicine and surgery was being practised at the home of the doctor or patient. The hospital was to take over this active role as the place for medical and surgical treatment during the nineteenth century. The older voluntary hospitals of London and those of the larger provincial towns increased in importance. Their own physicians and surgeons gradually assumed a teaching role, supplementing the traditional courses of the older universities and displacing the apothecaries and their apprenticeships.

The status of the surgeon significantly improved as he became recognised as a colleague of the physician on the hospital staff, where general competence in surgery or medicine was the desired attribute.

Long after the development of the specialties, it was the general physician and the general surgeon who held the top places in the hospital hierarchy. The 'senior surgeon' was always a general surgeon. Such attitudes led to the growth of separate specialist hospitals, which then attracted attacks from many general practitioners. Specialists were more to be feared as threats to incomes than were consultants. Patients could readily recognise under what heading their ailments came, and whether it was 'Eye' or 'Ear, Nose and Throat'. By passing the general practitioner, they might take themselves directly to the specialist concerned.

The demand arose for open access by all practitioners to hospital beds. The suspicions due to the conflicting interests of general practitioners and specialists prevented this from happening. Instead, the British system developed whereby all patients needful of a specialist's care, were first to be seen and then referred by a general practitioner. By this insistence it became firmly established that the patient 'belonged' to the general practitioner, even when removed to the care of a hospital specialist. The specialist's role was to advise the general practitioner on the care of his patient—advice which the general practitioner was free to accept or reject. This result was in the best interests of the patient, for whom his family doctor acted as a medical counsellor. A mutual respect grew up between the general practitioner and the consultant, whether of generic or specific type. It was nurtured by an intense loyalty felt by the doctor to his teaching hospital and teachers, which has lasted as a characteristic and tolerant affection until the present day.

THE CASUALTY OFFICER

Near the voluntary hospitals of the large towns patients sought the services of the casualty officer for their ailments. His service was usually good, easily available and free. In the nineteenth century, the local doctors felt cheated of their rightful fees and protested that the patients should consult them first, and be

3. SPLENDID OPENING FOR A YOUNG
        MEDICAL MAN (1848)

Chairman: 'Well, young man. So you
wish to be engaged as parish doctor?'

Doctor: 'Yes, gentlemen, I am
desirous—'

Chairman: 'Ah! Exactly. Well, it's
understood that your wages—salary
I should say—is to be twenty pounds
per annum; and you find your own
tea and sugar—medicines I mean—
and, in fact, make yourself generally
useful. If you do your duty, and
conduct yourself properly,
why—ah—you—ah—'

(*Punch:* 'Will probably be bowled out
of your situation by some humbug
who will fill it for less money.')

Reproduced by permission of Punch.

referred only if they felt it necessary (figure 2). When Robert Bridges, the poet laureate, was casualty physician at Bart's he had to examine, diagnose and prescribe for an average of 148 patients a morning. He found it as intolerable a burden as have many of his successors. The perennial problem of the overworked casualty physician brought the plea that there should be a limit to the number of cases expected to be seen by the honorary medical officer.

The British Medical Association of the time was concerned to keep the balance between the necessity for the health care of the 'deserving poor' and the reasonable income of its members. A means test was suggested as a more equable qualification for establishing the degree of poverty and controlling demand. Emergencies were to be dealt with on their medical merit alone. In 1904, the BMA Hospital Committee recommended that poverty and sickness should be the prime consideration for the admission of patients for hospital treatment.

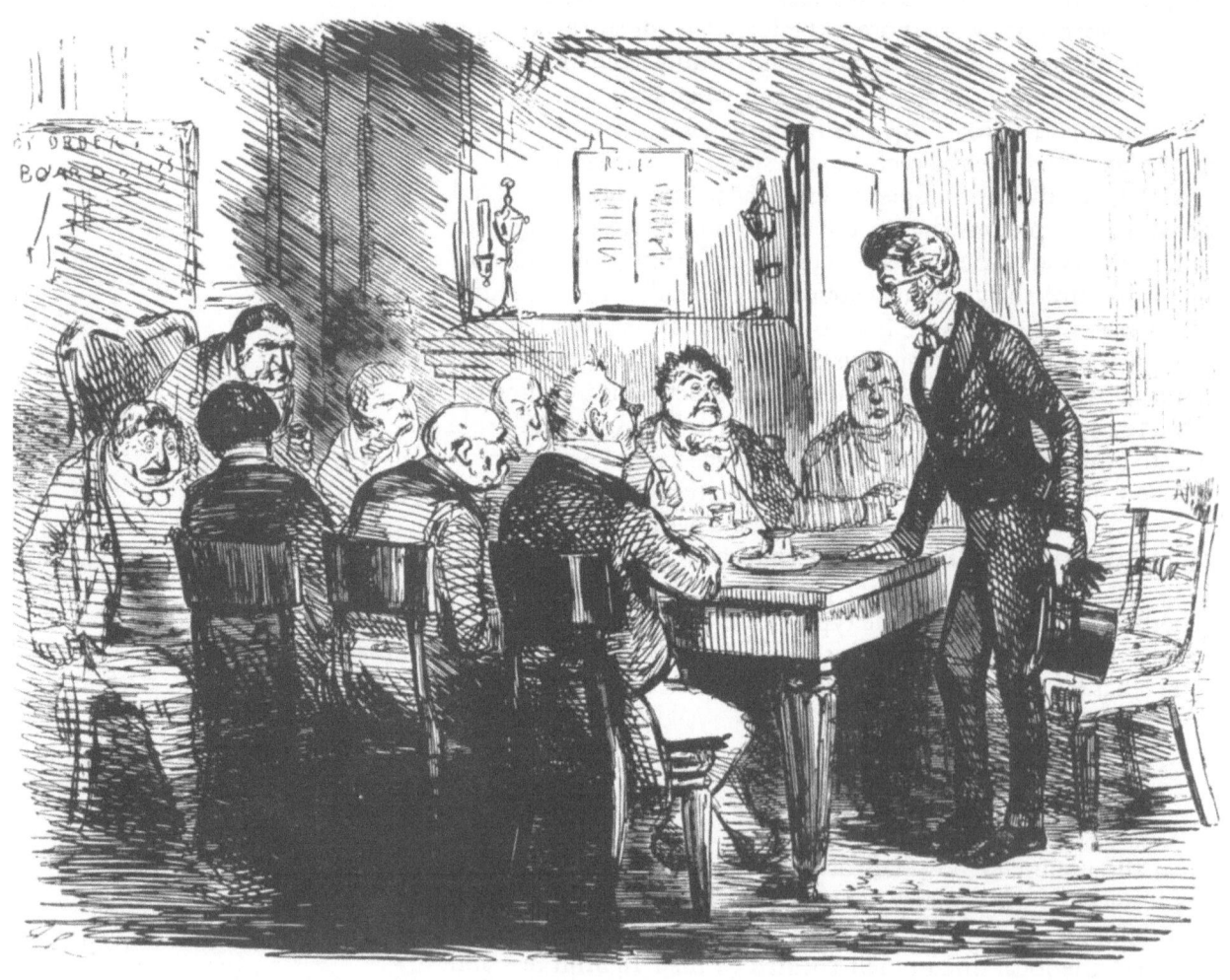

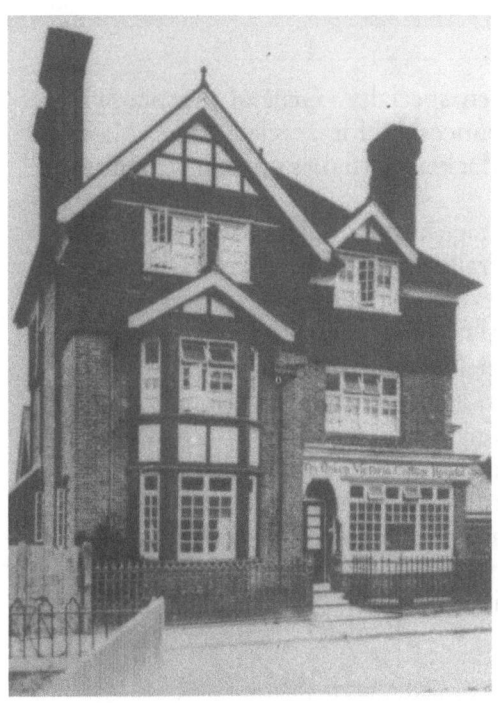
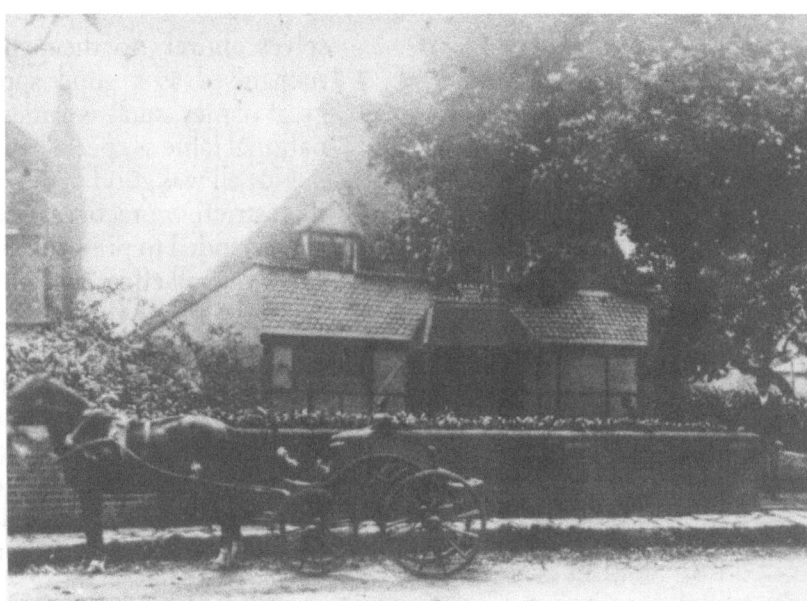

THE POOR LAW INFIRMARIES

The Poor Law infirmaries were yet other institutions whose fortunes were linked with those of general practice. The Poor Law medical officer, known as the 'parish doctor', was a grossly exploited practitioner, whose lowly status was related to his meagre pay (figure 3). He was employed by the Board of Guardians under very humiliating terms and was often expected to supply medicines from his own inadequate salary.

Before the 1858 Act the Poor Law medical officer was often only partly qualified and always poorly paid. As a result of pressures for the improvement of the infirmaries, described as State hospitals in work-house wards, the Poor Law Medical Officers Association encouraged the recruitment of a higher standard of doctors from the voluntary hospitals. The recruits were men who were unlikely to have succeeded in becoming appointed to the elite staff of the great hospital but whose aspirations lay elsewhere than general practice.

THE COTTAGE HOSPITALS

The general practitioner was usually excluded from any active role in the larger metropolitan hospitals, although in the country-side matters were different. Cottage hospitals (figures 4 and 5) where the general practitioner retained clinical control and management of his own patients, developed in the latter half of the nineteenth century. The facilities they provided attracted the active type of country practitioner to their areas and enabled them to practise a high standard of medicine and surgery.

Many general practitioners with special interests, fostered by their work in these hospitals, became recognised as specialists by their own colleagues, and whilst some developed these interests whilst remaining in general practice, others left to devote them-

4. The Queen Victoria Cottage Hospital, Queen's Road, 1907.
By courtesy of Dr E. J. Dennison.

5. Cranley Village Hospital, 1911. The original buildings of the first cottage hospital opened in 1859. The phaeton in the picture belonged to Dr A. A. Napper, the village doctor, son of the local surgeon, Mr Albert Napper, who was one of the founders of the hospital.
By courtesy of the League of Friends of Cranleigh Village Hospital.

selves entirely to their chosen specialty. General practice was recognised as a good apprenticeship for specialisation. Many great names, such as James Mackenzie (figure 6), achieved international fame as specialists.

Not all was good in the cottage hospitals. There were instances of restrictive practices, generally inspired by financial motives and intended to preserve the existing staff from new competition. Their overall effect on general practice was a good one and of the greatest value to the local patients whom they served.

The surgical side of the modern general practitioners' work later disappeared from its stronghold in the cottage hospitals after the inevitable acceptance and desirability of specialised surgery, which became so much more easily available after the National Health Service Act of 1946 came into force in July 1948 (figure 7). Until that time the general practitioner surgeon had maintained the only surgical service in many districts.

6. The Mackenzies in 1900.
   By courtesy of the Royal College of General Practitioners and Professor A. Mair.

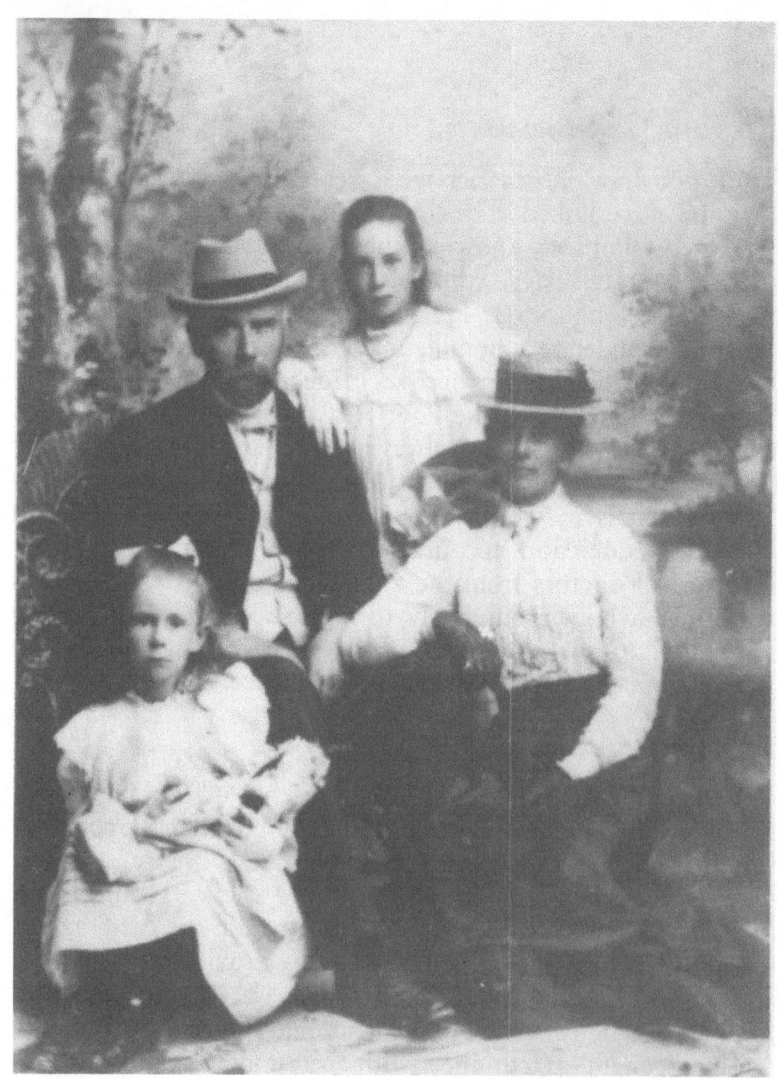

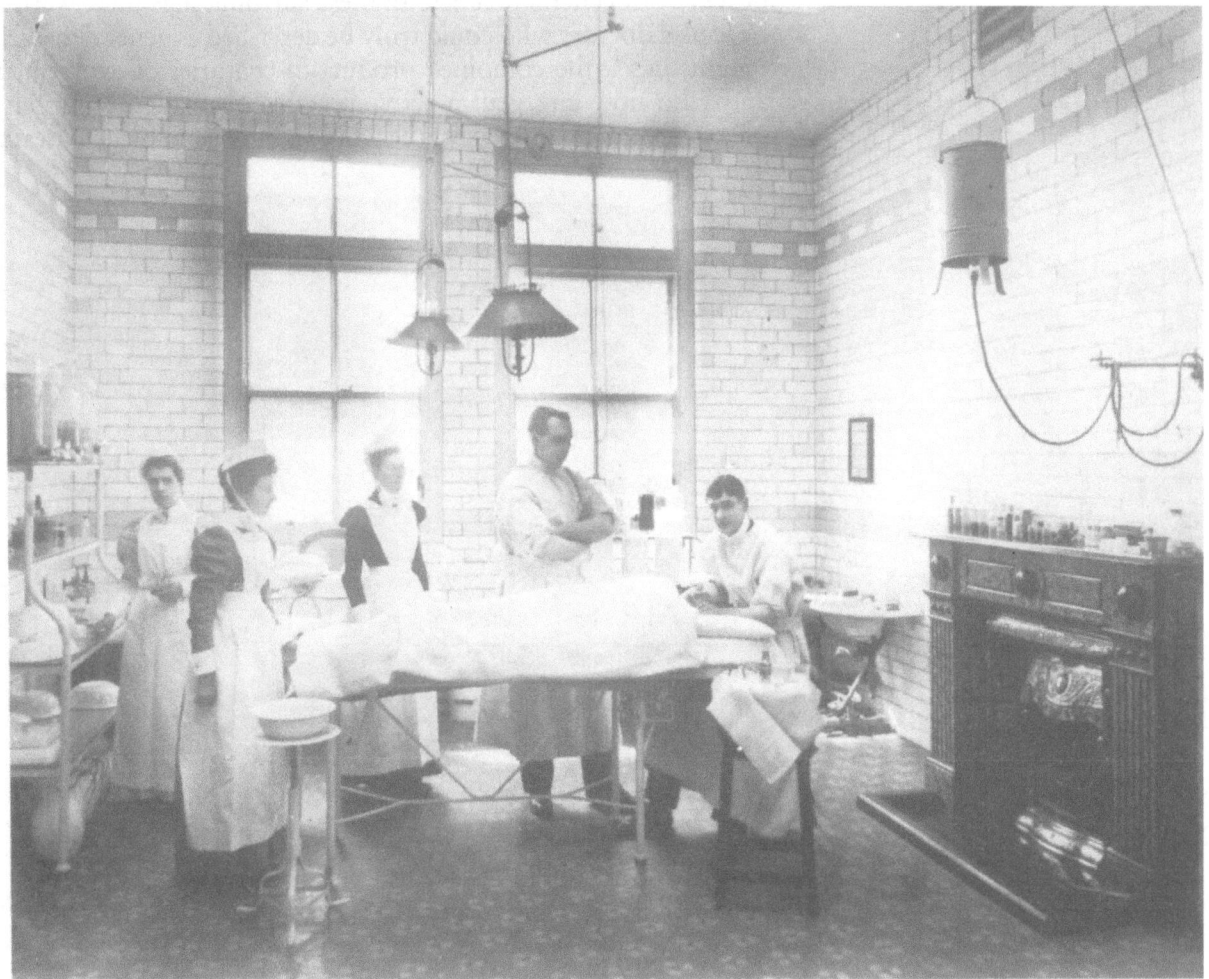

Toward the end of the nineteenth century, the general practitioner was recognisable as the modern family doctor (figures 8 and 9). By 1880, there were at least 180 cottage hospitals where he could give continuous care for his patients, in a pattern that was to remain largely unchanged until after Aneurin Bevan and William Beveridge.

Since then the idea of an adequately qualified, safe doctor fit to undertake any medical or surgical task, has become increasingly untenable. It was already under attack by the Flexner Report on Medical Education to the Carnegie Foundation in 1910. No longer was it possible to regard medical education as static—something one learned at medical school and which lasted a lifetime.

A scientific approach had to be taught, which would keep alive the student's interest through a medical career. The best general practitioners already did this for themselves, by taking part in medical societies which had flourished since the enthusiastic reformation of the nineteenth century. The fortunate ones were on the staffs of cottage hospitals, which had grown up in the second half of that century and provided the milieu for encouragement of the

7. The type of operating theatre in which the country general practitioner, who practised surgery and medicine, operated.

best type of general practice. In these surroundings there were to be found doctors who could truly be described as general medical practitioners, the combined product of centuries of evolvement and who now engaged in active practice of medicine, surgery, obstetrics and pharmacy for the whole family from birth to death.

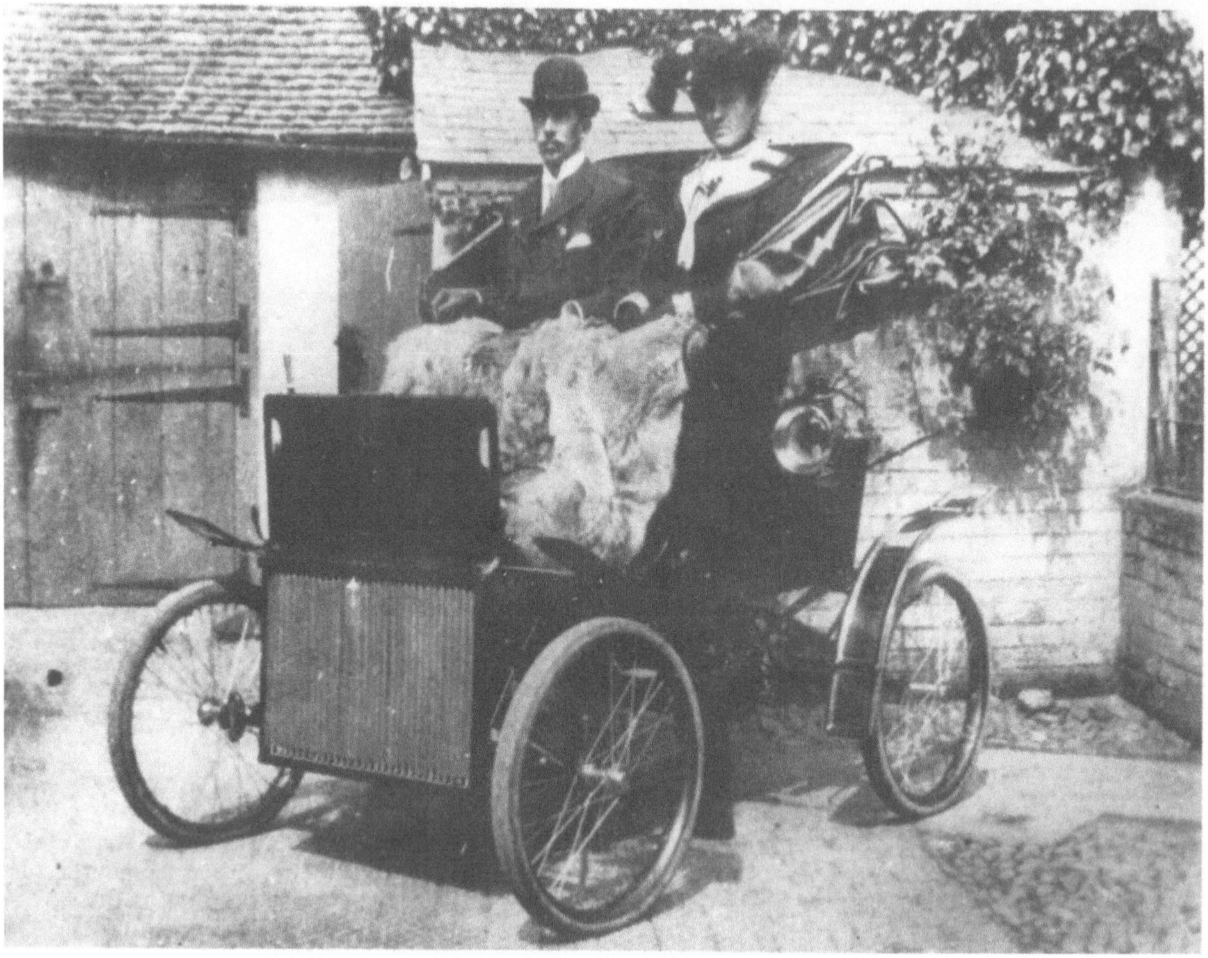

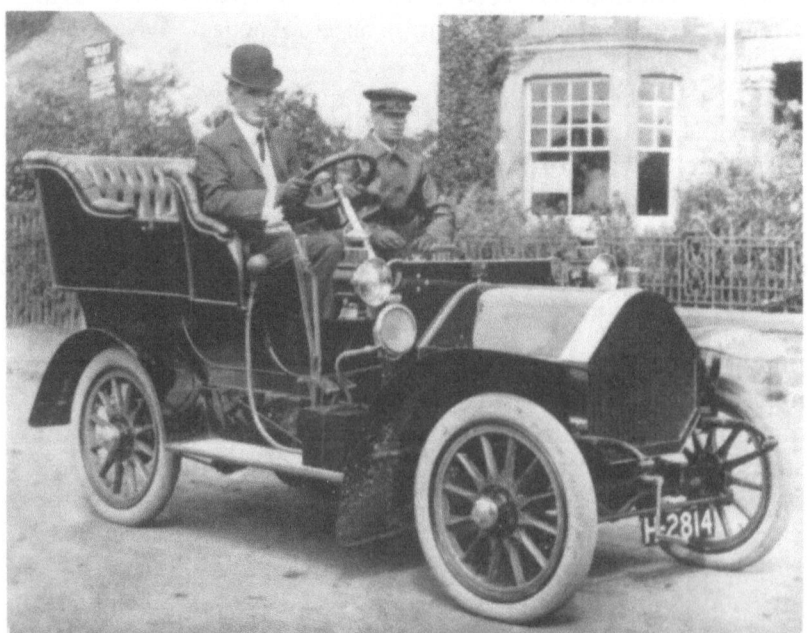

8. Dr and Mrs Tench in the stable yard in 1904, in a 'horseless carriage'.
By courtesy of Dr G. O. Barber.

9. Dr Harold M. Cooper, a general practitioner in Hampton-on-Thames from 1899–1929, on his rounds in 1906, in a 1905 Humber car.
By courtesy of Captain G. T. Cooper.

14
The National Insurance Act of 1911 and the State Medical Service

ATTITUDE TO THE POOR

Victorian attitudes encouraged individual thrift along with provision against hard times by savings with the friendly societies and provident clubs, that in many ways had taken over the charitable functions of the gilds. Poverty was regarded as a just punishment for indolence or iniquity (figures 1 and 2). The Edwardian upper classes, described as 'the supreme hedonists of British history', felt that the harsh conditions provided by the Poor Law actively discouraged people from sinking into poverty. The only virtue in charity was in its bestowal, not in its receipt. Those who accepted help under the Poor Law were regarded with shame. This forced the individual to do all he could to avoid the stigma of pauperism.

THE POOR LAW

Although the Poor Law was intended to provide care for the poor and deprived, its very name and its harsh application discouraged those in need of help. The Poor Law provided workhouse wards for sick paupers, and 'outdoor relief' with its dispensaries. The workhouse guardians, always anxious for financial economy, encouraged the development of independent sick clubs and provident dispensaries.

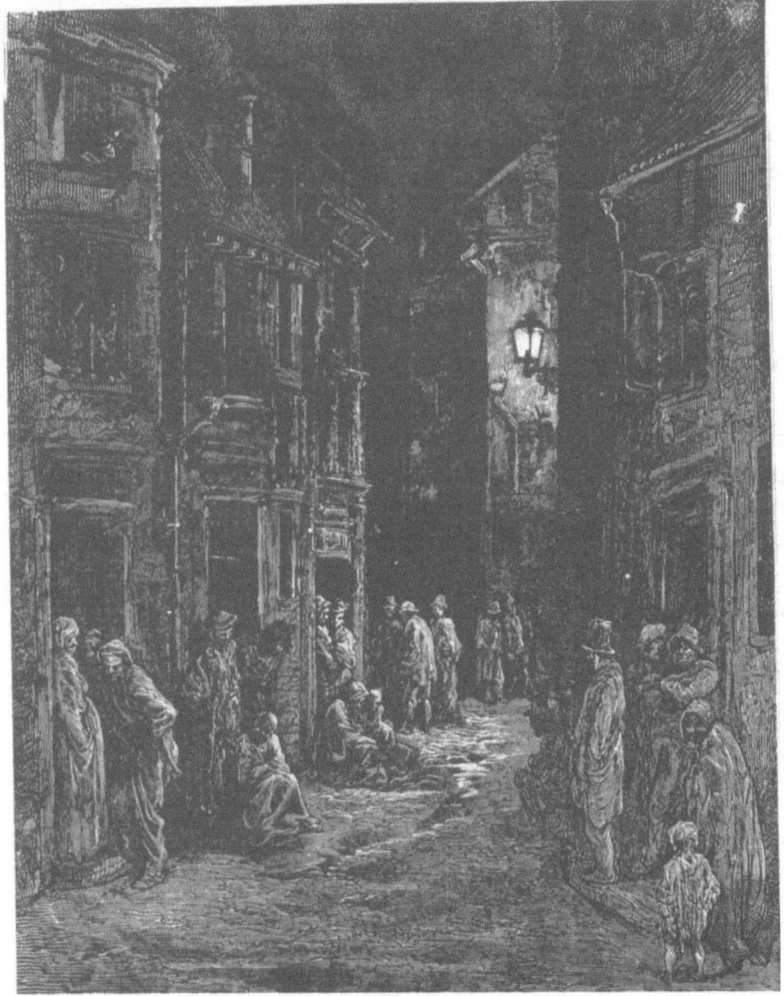

1. 'Bluegate Fields' by Gustav Doré. Doré was obsessed by the spectacle of human depravity. *Mary Evans Picture Library*.

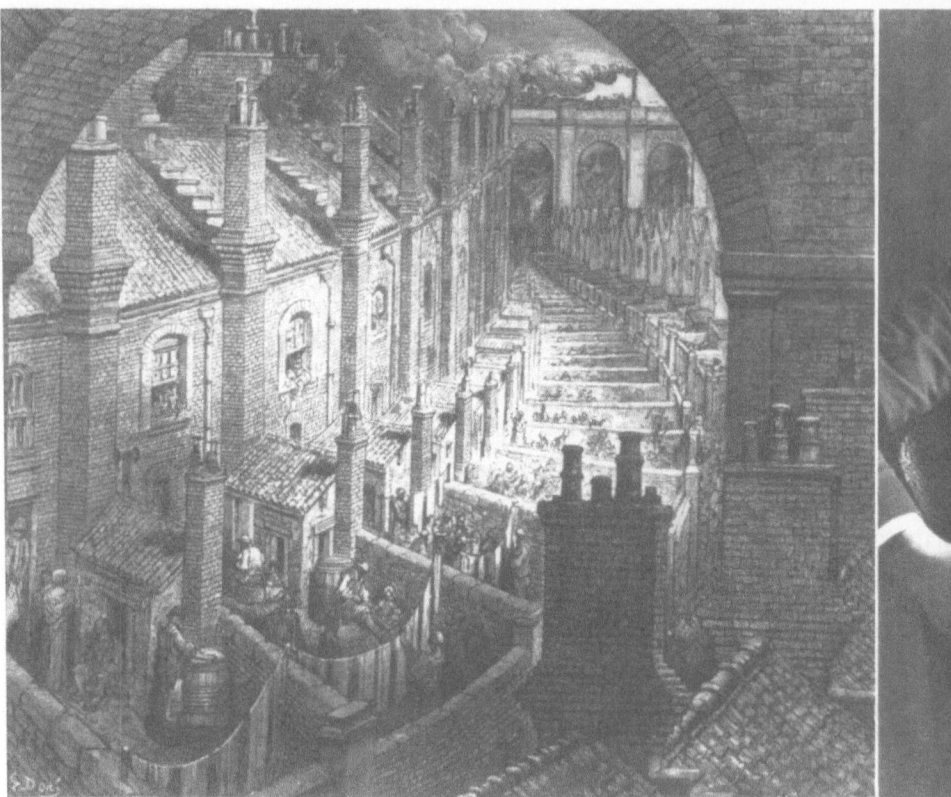
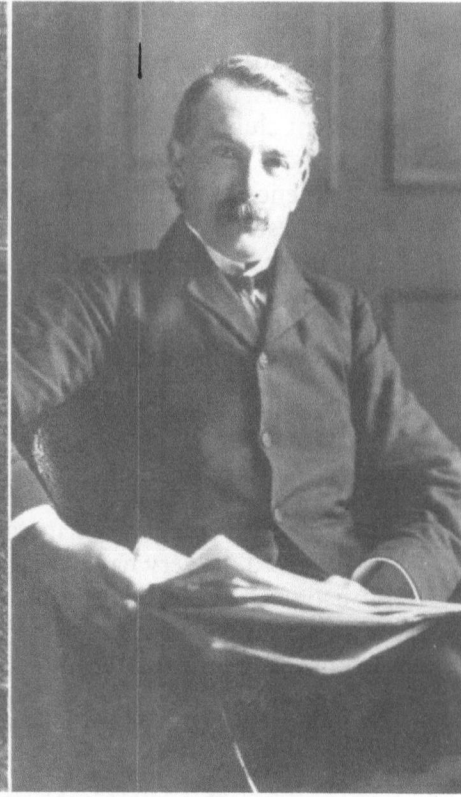

2. Slums under the railway bridge by
   Gustav Doré.
   Mary Evans Picture Library.

3. David Lloyd George in August 1908
   at Downing Street.
   BBC Hulton Picture Library.

PROVIDENT DISPENSARIES

Provident dispensaries were often controlled by wealthy patrons.
Working men and servants made small weekly contributions of
one or two pence, making them eligible for medical treatment.
Doctors on the staff were paid from the funds.

CONTRACT PRACTICE

The incomes of general practitioners with practices in working
class areas were largely dependent on the Poor Law guardians and
the committees of the medical provident clubs, as many of their
patients were themselves too poor to pay. The guardians were
notoriously mean and many doctors disliked working for the
provident clubs run by laymen who knew nothing about medicine.

Many friendly societies offered medical benefits during the
nineteenth century. Both they and the newer local medical clubs
employed doctors on a contract basis to provide care for their
members during illness, for a personal contribution of about four
pence a week. Contract practice was criticised because the doctors
provided an 'inferior' service, which they countered with the
excuse of 'inferior' pay.

Committees of both public and private aid institutions seemed
more interested in hiring cheap doctors to provide a cheap service
than they were in the quality or efficiency of medical care. They

paid their overworked doctors as little as possible. The committees of some private insurance schemes were the worst offenders; in order to make their annual premium fund as large as possible, they increased the number of subscribers well beyond the physical capacity of their underpaid medical servants.

In 1893 a special committee of the General Medical Council was set up to study these complaints. Its findings were published in a special 96 page Contract Practice Report Supplement to the *British Medical Journal* in 1905. The committee found it reprehensible for any doctor to:

1. hold a medical aid appointment the duties of which are so onerous that he cannot do justice to the sick under his care.

2. consent to give certificates where in his opinion they are not justified on medical grounds.

3. accept or retain employment by an association in which canvassing is used to attract members.

The General Medical Council did not take action on the recommendations of its committee.

A few medical clubs, run by the doctors themselves, managed to limit the amount of work to a level that gave their patients adequate medical care.

The National Health Insurance Act of 1911

THE NEED FOR STATE CONTROL

The British Medical Association was concerned about the control exercised over its members by the laymen in charge of provident schemes. It was to be a painful lesson that the mutual interests of both patients and doctors might best be met by government control of supply and demand.

Social reformers appreciated that poverty resulted from old age, sickness, death of the breadwinner and loss of jobs, as well as from fecklessness and personal inadequacy. In 1909 David Lloyd George (figure 3) had pledged his support for 'those who through no fault of their own are unable to earn their daily bread, the aged and infirm, the broken in health, the unemployed . . .'

The Old Age Pensions Act of 1908 had catered for the elderly, but did not help others who were unable to work. The 1911 Act was designed to assure the breadwinner against loss of income as a result of illness, unemployment (figure 4) or death.

THE ROLE OF THE FRIENDLY SOCIETIES AND INSURANCE COMPANIES

The National Insurance Act was not primarily a medical Act although it insured against the effects of sickness. The Treasury needed to take over the role of the friendly societies and commercial insurance companies. The insurance companies, such as

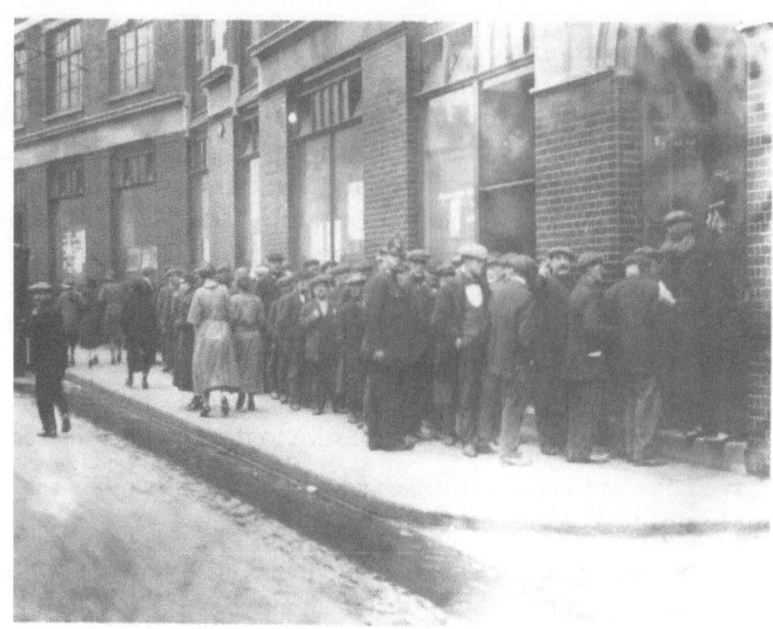

4. A queue waiting outside a labour
exchange, 1924.
BBC Hulton Picture Library.

the Prudential, were powerful political forces. They were in
regular contact with the working class and therefore could
influence public opinion for or against the Act. The takeover did
not prove difficult, however, when the capitalist insurance companies became 'approved societies' and were placed on an equal
footing with the friendly societies of radical tradition.

OPPOSITION TO THE ACT

The proposals put forward by the government placed the doctors
in a dilemma: they wanted to free themselves from the control of
the friendly societies, but they could now do this only through
state intervention, which they equally disliked. The BMA was
faced with the difficult task of trying to obtain the best possible
terms for its members.

On 1st June 1911, exactly four weeks after the introduction of
the Bill, the BMA presented Lloyd George with the 'Six Cardinal
Points':

1. An income limit of £2 a week for those entitled to medical
    benefit.

2. Free choice of doctor by patient, subject to consent of the
    doctor to act.

3. Medical and maternity benefits to be administered by insur-
    ance committees and not by friendly societies. In connection
    with the question of the method of administration of medical
    benefit, the Representative Meeting of the Association re-
    solved that all questions of professional discipline should be
    decided exclusively by a body or bodies of medical practi-

tioners, and that the power of considering all complaints against medical practitioners should be vested in a local Medical Committee, with a right of appeal to a central Medical Board to be appointed for that purpose.

4. The method of remuneration of medical practitioners adopted by each insurance committee to be according to the preference of the majority of the medical profession of the district of that committee.

5. Medical remuneration to be what the profession considered adequate, having due regard to the duties to be performed and other conditions of service.

6. Adequate medical representation among the insurance commissioners, in the central advisory committees, and statutory recognition of a local medical committee representative of the profession in the district of each insurance committee.

Through these proposals, the BMA expected to achieve professional control of the medical service, which would lead to more efficient organisation. The 'Six Cardinal Points' included improved pay and conditions of service for doctors, which in the BMA's view greatly influenced the quality of care.

THE AFTERMATH OF THE BILL

The Bill was introduced into Parliament on 4th March 1911 and after a stormy passage became law on 6th November. The provisions of the Act controlling medical benefits did not become operative until January 1913.

The BMA, however, asked all its members to sign an agreement not to work under the terms of the Act, until it had secured satisfaction on all six of its points. In January 1912, over 26,000 doctors out of a membership of 32,000, had signed and thus the sections of the Act dealing with insurance against sickness were rendered totally ineffective. Lloyd George adroitly managed to implement part of the Act in July 1912, without having to settle the question of doctors' remuneration, a major area of disagreement.

THE CAPITATION FEE

The method of payment eventually chosen by the doctors was by capitation fee, that is, a fixed sum for each registered patient 'on the panel'. A capitation fee of 6s (inclusive of drugs) had formed the basis of the actuarial calculations for the Act, but the BMA pressed for 8s 6d (exclusive of drugs). The BMA felt itself in a strong position because all members of the Association had been asked to sign an undertaking not to work under the terms of the Act, if they were not able to secure complete satisfaction on all six cardinal points.

The argument continued. Sir William Plender's Enquiry disclosed that the average capitation fee paid to doctors already in contract practice was 4s 2d, together with 3d for extras, and 5d for drugs, giving a total of 4s 10d. The Treasury was surprisingly persuaded to increase the proposed 6s, by a generous 50 percent, to a total of 9s. Despite the remarkable concessions of the government, a BMA meeting held on 21 December 1912, overwhelmingly rejected service under the Act and called upon its members to refrain from accepting office.

Contract doctors who were currently receiving less than half of the proposed capitation fee found the government's offer acceptable and many other members agreed. The BMA capitulated and reluctantly accepted what to everyone else seemed to have been the fruits of its resounding victory.

Beatrice Webb, of the Fabian Society, recognised that the Act had brought about a fundamental change in the structure of the medical profession:

The statutory constitution of the medical profession down to the passing of the National Insurance Act of 1911, consisted of the General Medical Council and its constituent elements—namely, the ancient medical

5. The health of many of the recruits for the Boer War was so poor that this highlighted the general ill-health of the population and increased pressure for public health reforms.
Mary Evans Picture Library.

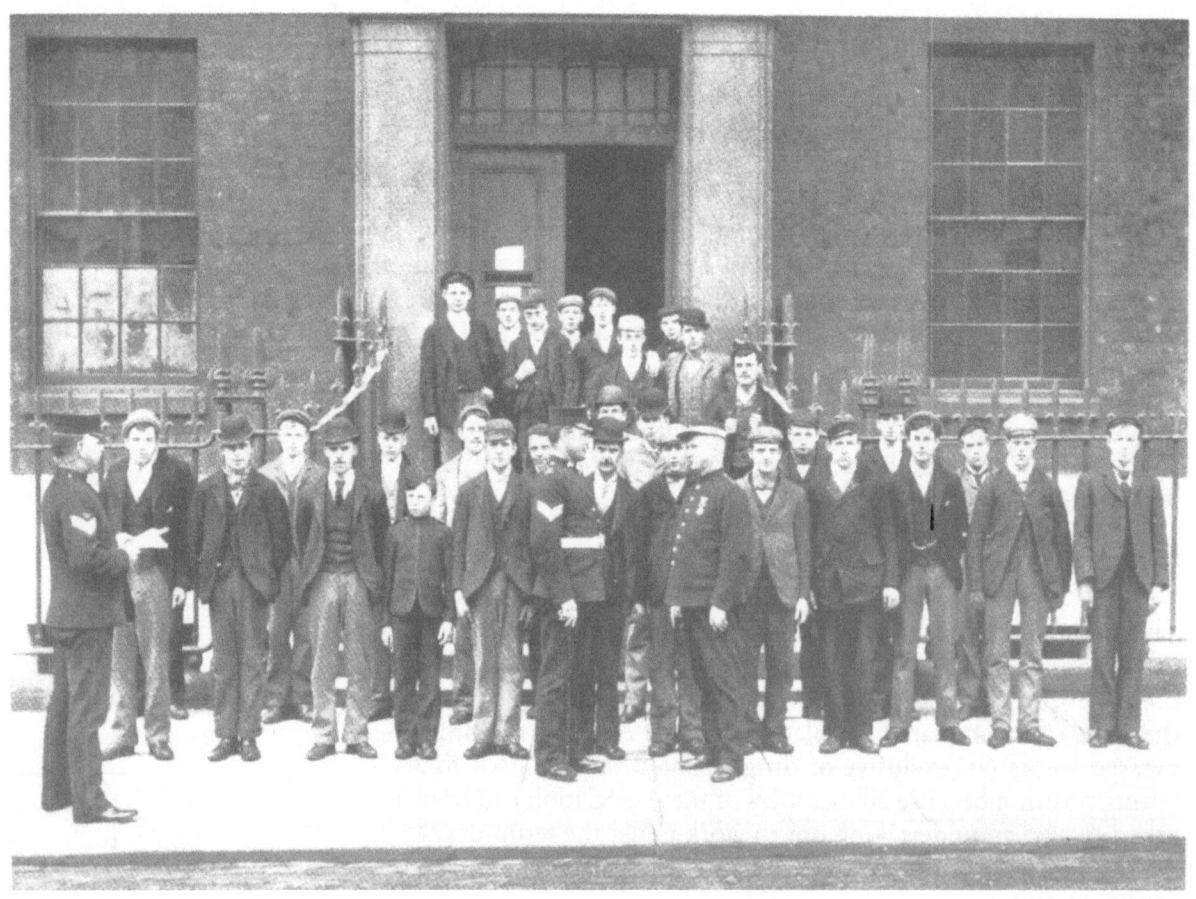

corporations, the old and new universities and the whole body of registered medical practitioners of the United Kingdom. The Insurance Act of 1911, for the purposes of medical benefit under that Act, set up a supplementary constitution for the profession.

The Implementation of the Act

THE HOSPITAL AND SPECIALIST SERVICE

The public health service and its sanitary reforms had been brought under state control in the nineteenth century (figure 5). The acute epidemics of cholera in the 1850s had ceased and given way to the chronic endemic disease of pulmonary tuberculosis by the early twentieth century. The Metropolitan Poor Act of 1867 had already created isolation hospitals for acute infectious fevers for which the illness of the patient and not his income had been the criterion for admission. The National Insurance Act of 1911 now established an anti-tuberculosis service with its specialist tuberculosis officer, 'the TO'. State and local authority combined in the building of sanatoria for hospital treatment. The Act of 1911 was amended to allow the Welsh local authorities to support the King Edward VII Welsh National Memorial Association for the prevention, treatment and abolition of tuberculosis. The Act also set up a school medical service for the early detection and prevention of disease in children (figures 6, 7, 8 and 9).

PRACTICE FINANCES

A general practitioner accepting service under the Act, received a capitation fee for each patient on his list, and in return he had to provide him with 'adequate treatment', as defined by the Act. Medical officers of the approved societies had the right to inspect the practitioner's patients and the treatment he gave them, and the doctor could be surcharged if his prescriptions were found to be extravagantly expensive.

General practitioners were no longer in competition with the outpatient departments of the hospitals as they had been at the end of the nineteenth century (see page 107). It was in the financial interest of some doctors to encourage patients to go to the hospitals for they had already received a capitation fee and did not get any extra payment for actual treatment. This tendency was more evident in large cities, and near large hospitals, rather than in the countryside where general practitioners played an important part in the running of the hospitals.

Although general practitioners were now represented on the insurance committees and local medical committees, they still had little control over their income, which was linked to the financial success or failure of the approved societies. The number of patients was as important as the capitation fee. All those people earning below £160 qualified at first for benefit under the 1911 Act, but

6. A head examination for lice at Chaucer Street School, 1911. *Greater London Council Photograph Library.*

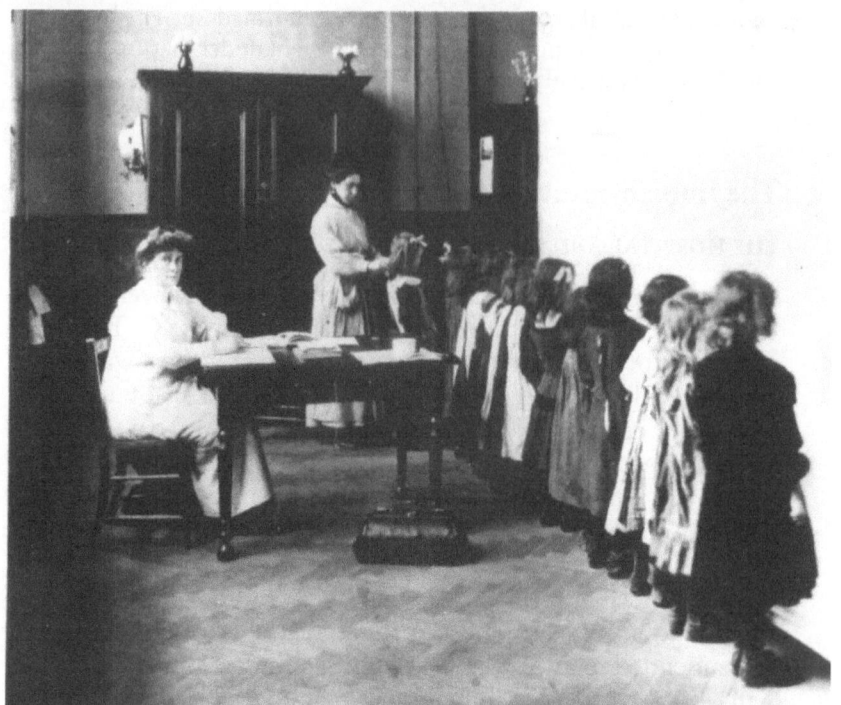

7. Finch Street Cleansing Station, 1911. Cutting verminous hair and sterilising clothes. *Greater London Council Photograph Library.*

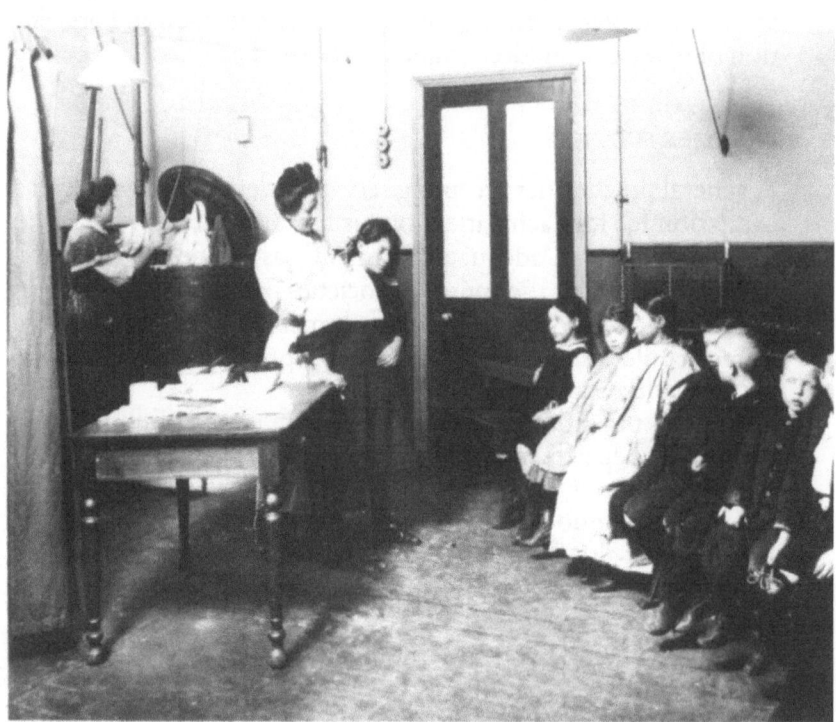

the effect of inflation, which followed the First World War, meant that the number of people eligible was greatly increased. The limit was raised to £250 in 1919, and it remained at this level until the Second World War.

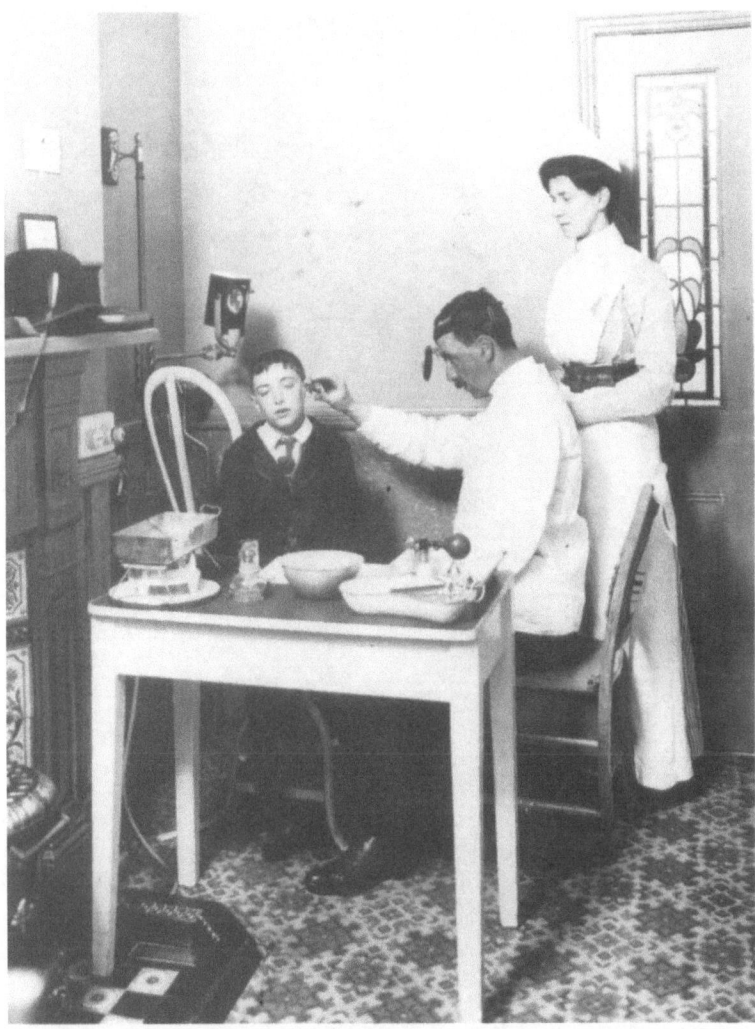

In the early 1920s, the general practitioners demanded that the capitation fee should be raised to 13s 6d. This was contested by the approved societies who believed that 7s 3d was ample. The two sides compromised on 11s, but after a financial crisis in 1922, the Ministry of Health reduced this fee to 9s 6d. The medical profession was greatly dissatisfied and the BMA was prepared to call a strike if necessary to improve remuneration.

Despite the complaints, the income of the average general practitioner had risen following the 1911 Act, and doctors could always supplement their state earned income with private practice. Private general practice flourished in middle class areas, where fee-paying patients often had their own separate entry to the surgery. Most working class patients felt that it was wise to seek a private consultation if they had anything more than a common ailment. They believed that they would receive better treatment if they paid for it. However, even in the 1920s the medical profession as a whole could still do little to cure serious illness, hence the maxim 'God heals but the Physician takes the fee'.

8. Ear examination at Wandsworth Medical Treatment Centre, 1911. *Greater London Council Photograph Library.*

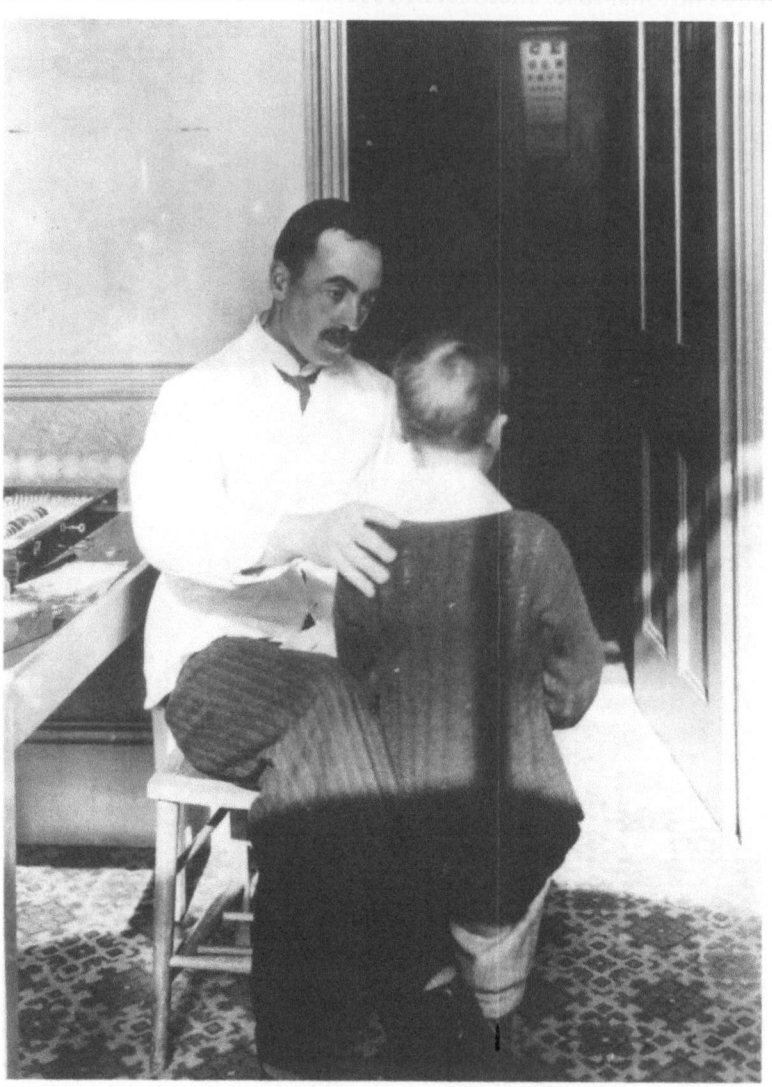

9. Sight testing at Wandsworth Medical
Treatment Centre, 1911.
*Greater London Council Photograph
Library.*

In working class areas the panel system became firmly established and associated with insurance certificates. The 'sick note'
became the distinctive mark of the panel and was of great importance to the patient.

The Therapeutic Revolution of the 1930s

In the first quarter of the twentieth century it mattered little how
soon the doctor made an accurate diagnosis, as there were hardly
any therapeutic measures he could use to cure specific illness. The
recovery of patients depended on good nursing, supportive care,
and the healing powers of nature. A doctor's reputation depended
on his knowledge of prognosis built on clinical experience, and on
his ability to offer comfort and reassurance. Although most of the
pills and potions available were of little pharmaceutical value,

they nevertheless played an important supportive role in treating ailments. Doctors were still taught how to roll pills and make up mixtures at medical school, even in the late 1930s when manufactured products had become widely available.

CHEMOTHERAPY AND ANTIBIOTICS

The foundations of chemotherapy were laid in 1904 when Paul Ehrlich (1854–1915) used 'Salvarsan' (arsphenamine) to treat syphilis. In 1935, Gerhard Domagk (1895–1964) published his discovery that 'prontosil' (sulphamidochrysoidin), a chemical compound of a sulphanilamide and a dye, was effective against streptococci. In 1937, it was shown that the active part was sulphanilamide, a member of the sulphonamide group, especially valuable in the treatment of some common and serious bacterial diseases (figure 10).

For the first time in medical history, it was no longer necessary to rely solely on nursing care in lobar pneumonia. The diagnosis of meningitis no longer meant certain death.

By 1940, Howard Walter Florey (1898–1969) and Ernst Boris Chain (1906–1979) had produced the antibiotic penicillin as a dry extract following the experimental discovery of Alexander Fleming (1881–1955) (figure 11) in 1929. Infectious diseases and fevers were conquered.

Scientists found that metabolic diseases could also be treated chemically. Frederick Banting (1891–1941) and Charles H. Best (1899–1978) (figure 12) discovered insulin in 1921. This immediately altered the prognosis of diabetes mellitus, and led to the manufacture of more sophisticated varieties of insulin such as protamine zinc insulin in 1936. The specialised treatment of diabetes meant a new life in place of invalidism for diabetics.

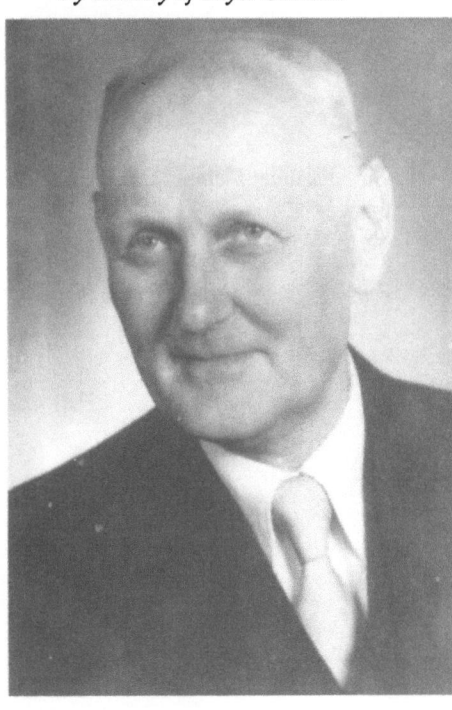

10. Professor Gerhard Domagk in 1894. *By courtesy of Bayer UK Ltd.*

The female sex hormones, discovered in the early 1930s, were made into an effective therapeutic tool with the synthesis of stilbestrol by Charles Dodds (1899–1973) (figure 13) and Robert Robinson (1886–1975).

THE EFFECTS OF THE THERAPEUTIC REVOLUTION

The therapeutic revolution changed the practice of medicine. The emphasis moved from the prevention of epidemic disease (figure 14) by public health reforms to the specific treatment of disease in the individual patient.

The pharmaceutical successes of the 1930s meant that diagnosis was no longer just a matter of academic and prognostic interest, but that early and accurate diagnosis was of prime importance in treating disease effectively. Enormous progress had been made but the concept of the generally qualified 'safe' doctor was still tenable and general practice was still considered a good training for later specialisation. It was possibly the last period when the medical curriculum, already alarmingly full, was not to be hopelessly overcrowded.

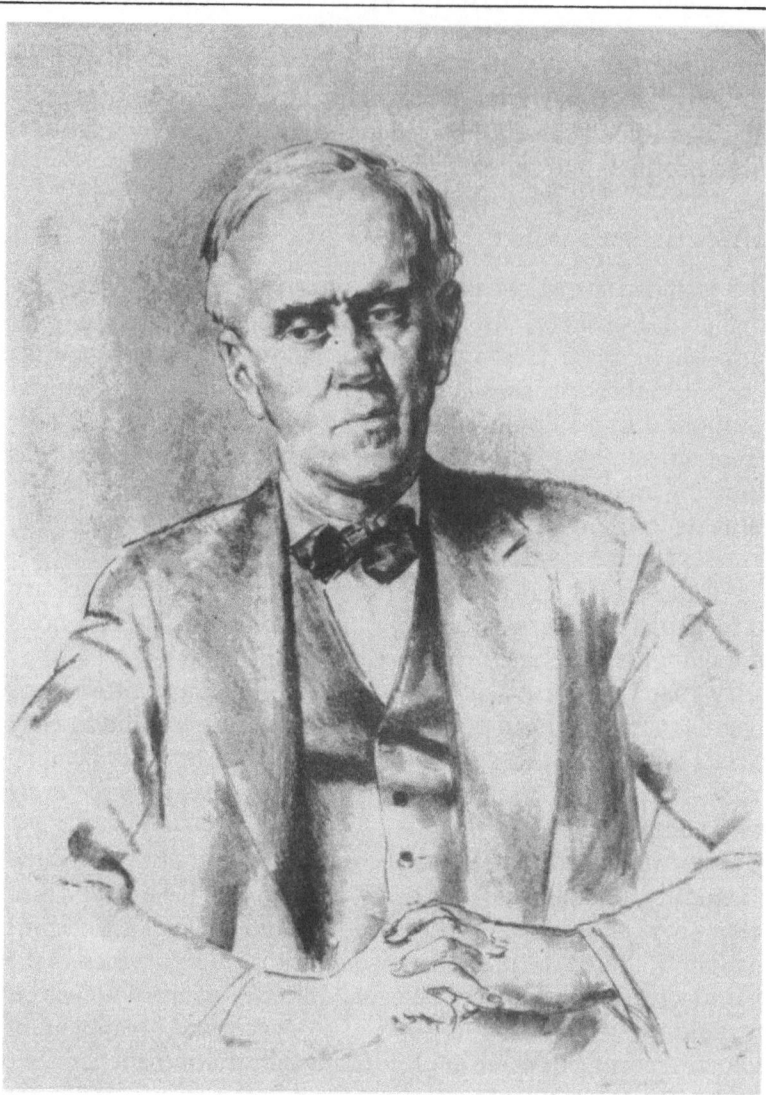

11. Sir Alexander Fleming, 1944, by
    J. A. Grant.
    *By courtesy of the National Portrait
    Gallery.*

The National Health Service

The Act of 1911 reduced the costs of medical attention for the insured breadwinner, but it did not provide any medical service whatsoever for his family. A financial cushion had been provided by the state for some members of society in times of illness. It was the beginnings of a state service but it was not a comprehensive national health service.

In 1834, a radical member of Parliament had denounced a proposal in support of a religious establishment, by comparing this with the 'ridiculous' idea of setting up a national health service:

You may as well propose a national medical establishment—and oblige everyone to pay for its support. Whether sick or well, all would then be called upon to pay the state physician.

By 1948 the climate of opinion had changed. The country had been united in fighting a common enemy, and had accepted many

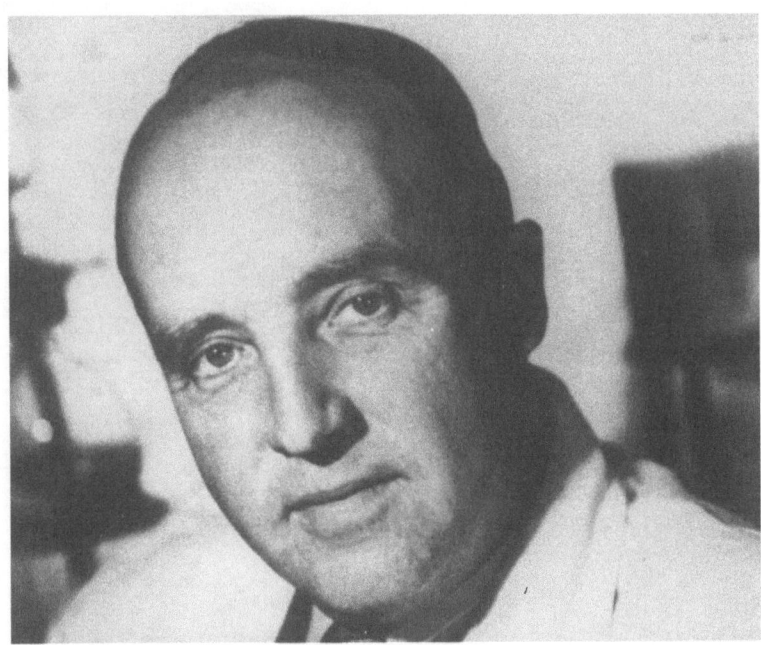

national establishments under state control. It was the Emergency Medical Service of the Second World War which firmly laid the foundations for the National Health Service Act of 1946. During the war, all citizens had been given a comprehensive hospital service, and all members of the armed forces had been given comprehensive primary medical care as well. A combination of these two would provide a national health service.

Many doctors in the EMS found it a surprisingly genial experience. For the generation of doctors who qualified during the war, the state services were their introduction to medicine and by the time it was over they were ready to accept the suggestions for a comprehensive national health service.

The 1946 Act met with initial hostility from the established medical profession. Many doctors felt that a contract with the state would interfere in the traditional doctor–patient relationship, and reduce the direct responsibility that the doctor felt for his patient. Not a few felt it would be a mortal blow to their professional liberty and status.

The theme and effect of the Act of 1858 had been one of unity. It stabilised a profession which had been torn apart by the power struggles of the apothecaries, surgeons and physicians. The Act of 1946 emphasised a disunity. It reflected the fragmentation of the profession caused by increasing specialisation. Some had even wanted to add a 'feldsher' class to relieve the lowest burdens of care from the NHS general practitioner.

Medical Qualifications

Today no qualification or licence is required in law for the practice of medicine in England and Wales, but no man who does so may

12. Dr Charles Best taken in the laboratory in 1948 by Rice and Bell for an article in Maclean Magazine. *By courtesy of the Banting and Best Department of Medical Research, University of Toronto.*

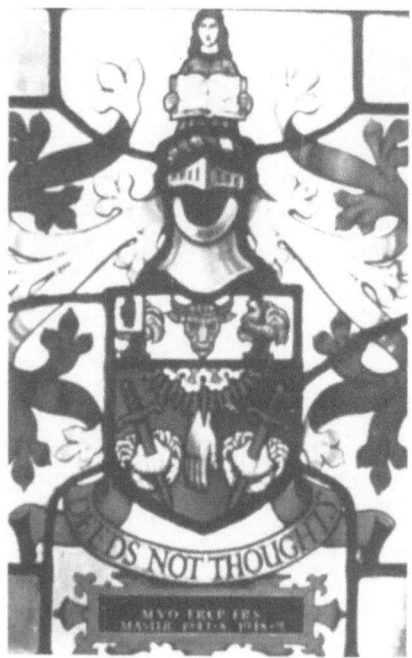

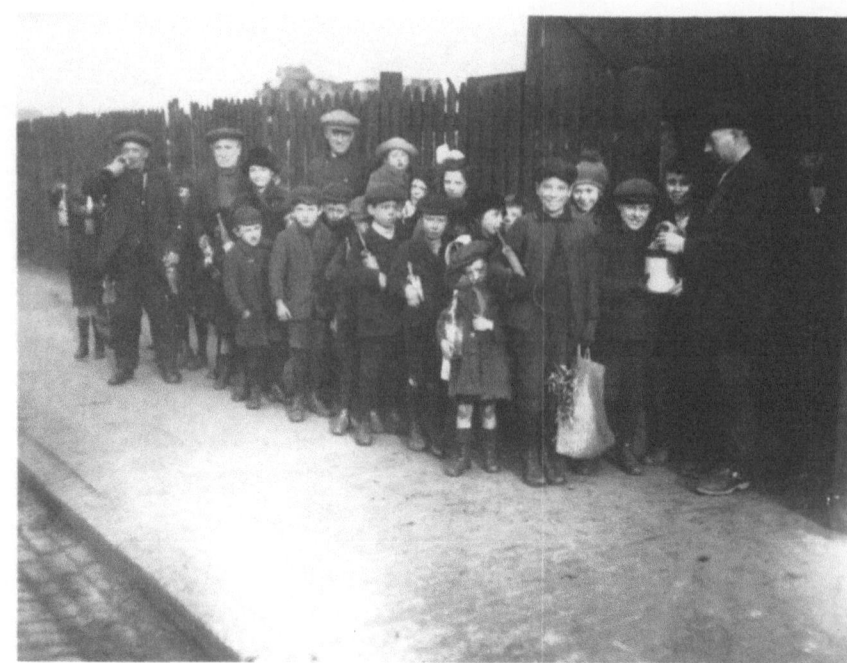

13. Memorial window to Sir Charles
    Dodds showing his coat of arms and
    formula for stilbestrol.
    *By courtesy of the Society of
    Apothecaries.*

14. A queue waiting for the distribution
    of 'flu fluid at Poplar, 1922.
    BBC Hulton Picture Library.

pretend that he holds a registrable qualification if he does not. Medical registration has enabled patients to distinguish between 'qualified' and 'unqualified' practitioners, and so to recognise whether or not they are competent.

Until 1953, registration required only the holding of a registrable qualification, but in that year the Medical Acts were amended to include a year of approved hospital appointments in general medicine and surgery as a compulsory pre-registration period after final examination. Apprenticeship has again been accepted as a requirement for all the profession.

The medical schools now require a student to take a university degree in medicine and surgery (MB, BS, or MB, B.CHIR) as his initial registrable qualification. The continued existence of the other registrable qualifications is at once a memorial to the inherent conservatism of the profession and the British reluctance ever to abandon a tradition.

The higher diplomas of the Royal Colleges, such as the Fellowship of the Royal College of Surgeons (FRCS), and Membership of the Royal College of Physicians (MRCP), are taken by postgraduates who wish to specialise in medicine or surgery. The higher degrees of the universities in medicine and surgery, are Doctor of Medicine (MD) and Master of Surgery (MS or M.CHIR). The specialties continue to multiply and when they receive the accolade of a Royal College they confer 'closed-shop' status on their members. Many hope that the Membership and Fellowship of the Royal College of General Practitioners will become the established requirements to mark the successful training for general practice.

The Medical Scientist

The growth of medical research and technology, outside strictly clinical medicine, has led to a new sort of doctor—a medical scientist, often but not invariably holding a medical degree. He makes an important contribution to diagnosis and treatment but is totally without a social function in relation to the patient. He is needed by the patient but may not even see him. He is essential to the progress of medical science, but works in a laboratory where his successes and failures are measured. His aspirations and rewards are not in the traditional terms of clinical skills and rewards.

The clinician himself may still have to rely on empiricism, on probability and on experience in making decisions. In this generation he may continue to have the sympathy of a laboratory colleague for these unfashionable qualities because they have shared a similar medical education. In the next generation time may not be available to train a man both as a clinician and a medical scientist. This will need a great reappraisal of relationships within the profession.

The relationship of technology to clinical care is not a new problem. Iatrophysicists of repute, like Giorgio Baglivi (1668–1706), the Italian who distinguished smooth and striped muscle, felt strongly that his sort of laboratory work did not help the patient. There is a ring of truth in his comment 'to frequent societies, to visit libraries, to own valuable unread books or shine in all the journals does not in the least contribute to the comfort of the sick'.

The devices of technology open a door but they do not compel one to enter. The dialogue between the technologist and the specialist also involves the patient and the general practitioner. Students who will become the technologists, the specialists, the patients and the general practitioners of the future may necessarily have to miss the unifying effects of a common medical education with its important humanitarian lessons.

Men are better doctors for an awareness of the wholeness of medicine in the common link which binds 'the body of physick'. Patients are happier for being treated as whole human beings rather than in their technical parts. A proper understanding of doctor–patient relationship in an age when medical science increasingly relies on the laboratory, depends on a proper understanding of the past.

Epilogue

The founding of the National Health Service seemed an appropriate point at which to end this book. The stage was already set for the New Therapy, which gave an even greater opportunity for change in medicine than that afforded by the New Learning of the Renaissance. The political climate was also ripe for the NHS Act to inaugurate a change in the financing of patient care. The general practitioner of the immediate pre-war era was to see a revolution in medical practice which would comprise a book in itself.

As we see, many of today's problems are not really new. Satisfactory medical care still requires more than technical knowledge. In the Tudor period competition between specialists for teaching time exposed the student to conflicting and confusing pressures and, even then, was a lively issue. Plantagenet preoccupation with an adequate supply of properly qualified doctors still exercises the managers of the National Health Service.

To see the patient as a whole human being requires a compassionate doctor, who is more often than not a man with a proper understanding of the past. History, moreover, helps one to remember the ephemeral nature of medical thought as we look at the many paths our predecessors took and enables us to evaluate the diagnostic improvements and therapeutic comforts that we enjoy today.

Further Reading

CHAPTER 1: PRE-ROMAN BRITAIN

Brothwell, D. R., *J. R. Anthropol. Inst.*, **91**, part 2. *Digging Up Bones.* London: British Museum, 1963.

Evans-Pritchard, E. E., *Social Anthropology*. London: Cohen & West, 1967.

Fleure, H. J., *A Natural History of Man in Britain*. London: Collins, 1951.

Ghalioungui, P., *Magic and Medical Science in Ancient Egypt*. London: Hodder & Stoughton, 1963.

Henschen, F., *The Human Skull*. London: Thames & Hudson, 1966.

Piggott, S., *Ancient Europe*. Edinburgh: Edinburgh University Press, 1965.

Sigerist, H. E., *A History of Medicine, Vol. I; Primitive and Archaic Medicine*. Oxford: Oxford University Press, 1967.

Wells, C., *Bones Bodies and Disease*. London: Thames & Hudson, 1964.

CHAPTER 2: ROMAN BRITAIN

Alcock, L. and Foster, I., *Prehistoric and Early Wales*, (Eds.) Foster, I. and Daniel, G. London: Routledge & Kegan Paul, 1965.

Brock, A. J., *Greek Medicine*. London: J. M. Dent & Sons, 1929.

Celsus, A. A. C., *De Medicina*, (Transl.) W. G. Spencer. London: Loeb Classical Library, 1961.

Garrison, F. H., *Notes on the History of Military Medicine*. Washington: Assoc. Mil. Surg., 1922.

Neuberger, M., *History of Medicine*, Vol I, (Transl.) E. Playfair. London: Frowde, 1910.

Richmond, I. A., *Roman Britain*. London: Pelican Books, 1964.

Richmond, I. A., *Univ. Durham Medical Gaz.*, 1952, June.

Singer, C., *From Magic to Science*. New York: Dover, 1958.

Webster, G., *The Roman Imperial Army*. London: Adam & Charles Black, 1969.

CHAPTER 3: THE ANGLO-SAXONS AND CELTS

Bede, *A History of the English Church and People*. Harmondsworth: Penguin, 1968.

Bonser, W., *The Medical Background of Anglo-Saxon England*. London: Wellcome Historical Medical Library, 1963.

Talbot, C. H., *Medicine in Medieval England*. London: Oldbourne, 1967.

CHAPTER 4: THE ANGLO-NORMANS

Matthews, L. G., *The Royal Apothecaries*. London: Wellcome Historical Medical Library, 1967.

Singer, C., *From Magic to Science*. New York: Dover, 1958.

Stenton, D. M., *English Society in the Early Middle Ages (1066–1307)*. Harmondsworth: Pelican History of England 3, 1969, 4th edition.

Talbot, C. H., *Medicine in Medieval England*. London: Oldbourne, 1967.

Talbot, C. H. and Hammond, A., *The Medical Practitioners in Medieval England. A Biographical Register*. London: Wellcome Historical Medical Library, 1965.

CHAPTER 5: THE LATER PLANTAGENETS

Cule, J., *J. of the Hist. of Med. and Allied Sci.*, 1966, 21: 213–236.

Matthews, L. G., *History of Pharmacy in Britain*. London: E. and S. Livingstone, 1962.

Myers, A. R., *England in the Late Middle Ages (1307–1536)*. Harmondsworth: Pelican History of England 4, 1963, 2nd edition.

Raach, J. H., *A Directory of English Country Physicians, 1603–43*. London: Dawsons, 1962.

Roberts, R. S., The personnel and practice of medicine in Tudor–Stuart England. *Medical History*, 1962, VI, 4: 363 and 1964, VIII, 3: 217.

Talbot, C. H., *Medicine in Medieval England*. London: Oldbourne, 1967.

Talbot, C. H. and Hammond, E. A., *The Medical Practitioners in Medieval England. A Biographical Register*. London: Wellcome Historical Medical Library, 1965.

CHAPTER 6: THE TUDORS

Roberts, R. S., *Medical History*, 1962, VI, 4: 363 and 1964, VIII, 3: 217.

Talbot, C. H. and Hammond, E. A., *The Medical Practitioners in Medieval England. A Biographical Register*. London: Wellcome Historical Medical Library, 1965.

CHAPTER 7: THE THEORY AND PRACTICE OF TUDOR MEDICINE

Holmyard, E. J., *Alchemy*. Harmondsworth: A Pelican Original, 1968.

Withington, E. T., *Medical History*. London: The Holland Press, 1964.

CHAPTER 8: THE STUARTS

Cope, Z., *Brit. Med. J.*, 1956, 1: 1.

Copeman, W. S. C., *Brit. Med. J.*, 1967, 4: 540.

Forbes, T. R., *Chronicle from Aldgate, Life and Death in Shakespeare's London*. New Haven and London: Yale University Press, 1971.

Foster, M., *Lectures on the History of Physiology during 16th, 17th and 18th Centuries*. New York: Dover Press, 1970.

Keynes, G., *The Life of William Harvey*. Oxford: Clarendon Press, 1966.

Raach, J. H., *A Directory of English Country Physicians 1603–1643*. London: Dawsons, 1962.

Whittet, T. D., *Medical History*, 1964, VIII, 3: 245.

CHAPTER 9: THE HOUSE OF HANOVER

Cope, Z., *A History of the Royal College of Surgeons of England*. London: Anthony Blond, 1959.

McConaghey, R. S., *The Evolution of Medical Practice in Britain*, (Ed.) Poynter, F. N. London: Pitmans, 1961.

Young, S., *The Annals of the Barber-Surgeons of London*. London: Blades, East and Blades, 1890.

CHAPTER 10: THE APOTHECARIES ACT OF 1815

Holloway, S. W. F., *Medical History*, 1966, 10, 3.

Matthews, L. G., *History of Pharmacy in Britain*. Edinburgh and London: E. and S. Livingstone, 1962.

CHAPTER 11: NINETEENTH CENTURY EDUCATIONAL REFORM OF GENERAL PRACTICE

Christison, R., *The Life of Sir Robert Christison*, (Ed. His sons). Edinburgh and London: W. Blackwood & Sons, 1885.

Cope, Z., *The History of the Royal College of Surgeons of England*. London: Anthony Blond, 1959.

Holloway, S. W. F., *Medical History*, 1966, 10, 3.

Brotherston, J., *Medical History and Medical Care*, (Eds.) McLachlan, G. and McKeown, T. Oxford: Oxford University Press, 1971.

Rivington, W., *The Medical Profession*. Dublin: Fannin & Co., 1879.

Thornton, J. L., *John Abernethy*. London: Simpkin Marshall, 1953.

CHAPTER 12: THE MEDICAL ACT OF 1858

De Styrap, J., *The Young Practitioner*. London: H. K. Lewis, 1890.

Lambert, R., *Sir John Simon: 1816–1904*. London: McGibbon & Kee, 1963.

Newman, C., *The Evolution of Medical Education in the Nineteenth Century*. Oxford: Oxford University Press, 1957.

Rivington, W., *The Medical Profession*. Dublin: Fannin & Co., 1879.

CHAPTER 13: VICTORIAN MEDICINE

Ashe, I., *Medical Education and Medical Interests*. Dublin: Fannin & Co., 1868.

Brotherston, J., *Medical History and Medical Care*. (Eds.) McLachlan, G. and McKeown, T. Oxford: Oxford University Press, 1971.

Osler, W., *Boston Med. Surg. J.*, 1892, **126**: 457–459.

St Bartholomew's Hospital Reports, 1878, **14**: 167.

White, L., *Medieval Technology and Social Change*. Oxford: Oxford Paperbacks, 1962.

CHAPTER 14: THE NATIONAL INSURANCE ACT OF 1911 AND THE STATE MEDICAL SERVICE

Brand, J. L., *Doctors and the State*. Baltimore: Johns Hopkins Press, 1965.

Davies, J., *Wales and Medicine*, (Ed.) Cule, J. Llandysul: British Society for the History of Medicine, 1975.

Jones, G. R., *Wales and Medicine*, (Ed.) Cule, J. Llandysul: British Society for the History of Medicine, 1975.

Little, E. M., *History of the British Medical Association 1832–1932*. London: B.M.A., 1932.

Parry, Noel and José, *The Rise of the Medical Profession*. London: Croom Helm, 1976.

White, L., *Medieval Technology and Social Change*. Oxford: Oxford Paperbacks, 1962.

Index

Index

Index

Index

Index

Index

Index